How Does Analysis Cure?

Building upon 50 years of clinical experience, Fred Busch addresses a central question facing all psychoanalysts: What is essential to a psychoanalytic curative process, and what are the methods of working that can bring this about?

This book investigates the analytic relationship as a process of giving patients the freedom to think the unthinkable (to build representations) and change repeated patterns of action into the possibility of reflection. This entails careful examination of central psychoanalytic concepts such as transference, resistances, and the ethics of countertransference as a guide to a patient's unconscious, in addition to newer ideas, such as the notion of the analyst as a memory keeper of patients' lost objects. In its final part, the book presents observations on how analysts function as part of analytic organizations, and the various roles they take on to develop an "analytic identity".

Continuing decades of significant theoretical work on clinical concepts, this book offers a unique perspective on how psychoanalysts and psychotherapists can work effectively to achieve the best possible outcomes for their patients.

Fred Busch, PhD, is a training and supervising psychoanalyst at the Boston Psychoanalytic Institute. He has published 8 books and over 80 articles on psychoanalytic technique. Most recently, he wrote *A Fresh Look at Psychoanalytic Technique,* and he is editor of *Psychoanalysis at the Crossroads* and *The Ego and Id: 100 Years Later* (with Natacha Delgado).

W0113332

'With his unmistakable sharp and essential style, Fred Busch takes us on a high-quality free-thinking experience of contemporary psychoanalysis, theoretical-clinical research, fundamental concepts such as free association, the preconscious and action language, and the priceless 'being in the neighbourhood', as well as institutional processes and training for a profession as special as ours.

Maintaining an enviable critical and self-analytical serenity, Busch cultivates a natural, genuine curiosity towards the contributions of his colleagues, which then leads him to formulate his own complex, documented, finely thought-out and well-integrated vision of the analytical events on display. An extraordinary book by a true analytical mind.'

Stefano Bolognini, *IPA past-president, training and supervising analyst, Italian Psychoanalytic Society, Bologna, Italy*

'In this thoughtful book, the prolific psychoanalytic author, Fred Busch, contributes another chapter in his ongoing exploration of a contemporary Freudian perspective on a theory and technique of psychoanalytic treatment. Busch is one of our clearest thinkers, with a wide-ranging knowledge of multiple perspectives. This allows him to compare and contrast his view with other theories of technique, always in a respectful manner. The first two chapters of this book capture the essence of his views on how analysis cures. This is followed by a series of chapters where Busch explores clinical issues, like transference, and finds new meaning in them. In the second section of the book Busch raises issues about our profession that are rarely explored (ex., The Gossip, The Good-Enough Discussant, etc.). In short this is a book, along with *Creating a Psychoanalytic Mind*, that needs to be read and studied.'

Virginia Ungar, *past IPA president, training and supervising analyst, Buenos Aires, Argentina*

How Does Analysis Cure?

Essays on a Psychoanalytic Method,
Psychoanalytic Organizations and
Psychoanalysts

Fred Busch

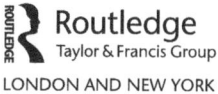
Routledge
Taylor & Francis Group

LONDON AND NEW YORK

Designed cover image: © OsakaWayne Studios / Getty Images.

First published 2025
by Routledge
4 Park Square, Milton Park, Abingdon, Oxon OX14 4RN

and by Routledge
605 Third Avenue, New York, NY 10158

Routledge is an imprint of the Taylor & Francis Group, an informa business

British Library Cataloguing-in-Publication Data
A catalogue record for this book is available from the British Library

ISBN: 978-1-032-65872-8 (hbk)
ISBN: 978-1-032-65868-1 (pbk)
ISBN: 978-1-032-65870-4 (ebk)

DOI: 10.4324/9781032658704

Typeset in Sabon
by Deanta Global Publishing Services, Chennai, India

Note on the Cover Image

The psychoanalytic cure is a "consequence of the analyst helping the weakened ego, giving it back *its mastery over lost provinces of his mental life.*"

Freud (1940). An Outline of Psycho-Analysis. *International Journal of Psychoanalysis* 21:27–84.

A Parable for a Psychoanalytic Cure

Recently I read a newspaper article about a Mr. Woodfox, age 69, who was in prison for 45 years, most of the time in solitary confinement. When he was released from prison, he was asked what it was like to be in solitary confinement for so long. His answer serves as the basis of what I consider curative in psychoanalysis. He said, *"When I began to understand who I was, I considered myself free."* He added, *"No matter how much concrete they used to hold me in a particular place they couldn't stop my mind."*

Routledge Books by Fred Busch

Creating a Psychoanalytic Mind: A Psychoanalytic Method and Theory (2013)

The Analyst's Reveries: Explorations in Bion's Enigmatic Concept (2019)

Dear Candidate: Analysts from Around the World Offer Personal Reflections on Psychoanalytic Training, Education, and the Profession (F. Busch, editor, 2020)

A Fresh Look at Psychoanalytic Technique: Selected Papers (2021)

Psychoanalysis at the Crossroads: An International Perspective (F. Busch, editor, 2023)

The Ego and the Id: 100 Years Later (F. Busch & N. Delgado, editors, 2023)

I dedicate this book to my wife and colleague, Cordelia Schmidt-Hellerau, whose help and support has widened my horizons and enriched my life. Also, my special thanks to Cecilio Paniagua, who helped me find answers to unformulated questions and remains my good friend and wise critic.

Contents

Acknowledgments

Chapter 7 first appeared in the *Scandinavian Psychoanalytic Review:* Busch, F. (2021). Self-criticism as an unconscious lifeline. *Scandinavian Psychoanalytic Review* 44:20–26.

Chapter 18 first appeared in the *International Journal of Psychoanalytic Controversies:* Busch, F. (2020). The troubling problem of authority in psychoanalytic institutes. *Int. J. of Controversial Discussions* 2:3–26.

Introduction

After reading various articles on the analyst's character and its effect on how he analyzes, I spent time reflecting on how my character might have played a role in how I analyze. I could see elements of it, but I believe such formulations applied in a global fashion can leave out the important part that theory, supported by data, can play in evaluating different theories. Upon reflection, I could see how my graduate training in psychology primed me to think like a researcher when evaluating different psychoanalytic approaches. I believe that my technique is primarily rooted in my pre-analytic training, in the works of Heinz Hartmann, David Rapaport, and my post-doctoral training experience where we intensively studied the work of Anna Freud, led by analysts trained at the Hampstead Clinic (later called The Anna Freud Center). In these centers, the ego and how it functioned was an important topic.[1] When newer theories became part of the psychoanalytic landscape during my analytic training (e.g., Kohut, object relations, and developmental theory), I could understand their relevance based on my earlier experiences of working psychotherapeutically with children and observations of nursery and toddler groups for many years.

At the time of my pre-analytic training as a psychologist, I did a lot of psychological testing. In my clinical internship, my post-doctoral fellowship, and my first university appointment, I gave hundreds of psychological tests that consisted of projective tests (i.e., Rorschach, Thematic Apperception Test) and an intelligence test. My testing supervisors in my pre-doctoral internship were trained at Menninger according to the Rapaport, Gill, and Schafer (1945) method, where their revolutionary approach focused on the *form of thinking* rather than the *content* alone. In this way, one could differentiate neurotic disturbances from the more severe *character disorders* based on ego functioning. Other professionals would make referrals based on trying to find out if the patient was in the Oral, Anal, Phallic, or Oedipal stage,[2,3] when the underlying questions had to do with differentiating the neurotic patient from the borderline or psychotic in terms of suitability for treatment. *In short, the underlying question the referring person was asking had to do with a diagnosis of the degree of intactness of the patient's ego.* Thus, I was trained early on to look not

DOI: 10.4324/9781032658704-1

only at the content of what patients thought, but possibly even more important was to also evaluate *how a patient thought about what they thought about*, which focused on their ego functioning. Previous models of understanding the Rorschach were based on content alone.

In a continuing refrain throughout his work, Rapaport emphasized the importance of *thinking about thoughts*. His major contribution was expressed this way: "Though the understanding of *content* is sufficient for everyday communication and for many needs of diagnostic and therapeutic practice, it is insufficient for understanding of personality and thought processes. *Consideration of contents will have to be supplemented and reinterpreted into formal characteristics of the thought process*" (1951/1967, pp. 432–434, italics added). This perspective has been evident in all my work since the early 1990s. Yet, throughout my pre- and post-doctoral training, along with my analytic training, it was a puzzle how these concepts could be applied to clinical psychoanalytic work. My search was complicated because in my psychotherapy and psychoanalytic training, we were primarily taught to pay attention to the *content* of what patients were revealing. Interpretations were mostly based on content alone. It was striking to me that although my Institute was known as an ego-psychological institute, immersed in the work of Arlow and Brenner, there was little attention paid to the ego.[4] It was only later that I realized that Arlow and Brenner eschewed some basic principles of their predecessors at the New York Psychoanalytic Institute (Hartmann, Kris, and Lowenstein) who were pioneers in developing ego psychology. This became obvious when Brenner (1982) stated that there are no separate agencies in the mind (id, ego, super-ego), only compromise formations, thus negating Freud's second model of the mind. So, I spent much of my analytic training making deep interpretations, which my patients reacted to with indifference, at best, but also with resentment. I only realized later that I was bypassing defenses which led the patient to feel "found out".

I have written previously (Busch, 2013) how my epiphany came at the meetings of the International Psychoanalytic Association in Barcelona, Spain, where I heard a colleague (Cecilio Paniagua) respond to a paper in a way that reflected what I was struggling to articulate. He mentioned the work of Paul Gray and his 1982 paper on a developmental lag in technique, which started me on my 30-year journey to articulate a method of psychoanalytic treatment focused on the role of the ego. While I followed Paul Gray's method of working for about 10 years, I eventually found it to be somewhat restrictive,[5] and started to find new ways of working that helped patients discover the stories they never knew that drove them and helped them to find their own mind (Busch, 2013, 2015).

Essential to my growth as an analyst was the gentle nudging of my wife, Cordelia Schmidt-Hellerau, to branch out and read more of the literature from Europe, which helped me to broaden my outlook and find a certain kinship with the thinking of Pierre Marty and the Paris Psychosomatic School (Aisenstein, 2014; Aisenstein and Smadja, 2010). In his ground-breaking work, Marty discovered it was a particular way of thinking (concrete), and thinking without thoughts, that characterized psychosomatic patients' mental processes. Thus, with this type of patient, it was understanding the *characteristics of their thinking*, not the content alone, as championed by Franz Alexander (1965), which dominated the thinking of North American psychoanalysts for many years. As one can see, Marty's perspective fit well with my own growing understanding of the necessity of the analyst's focus of attention on the patient's way of thinking along with the content of their thoughts. Andre Green's (1974, 1975) early writing about the importance of the preconscious in the interpretive process led me to focus more on what was *potentially preconscious* (Busch, 2006, 2013) rather than what was conscious in my interpretations. Finding commonality with certain Latin American analysts' (e.g., Elias and Elizabeth de Rocha Barros, and Roosevelt Cassorla) was an exciting discovery.

After years of observing children in my post-doctoral training and my first academic position, I became interested in the work of Jean Piaget and his views on the development of children's thought processes, which was invaluable in my understanding of what I called *language action* (Busch, 1995, 2009, 2013), and the concrete thinking of certain patients.

This book is a continuation of my previous book, *Creating a Psychoanalytic Mind (2013); together they serve as an attempt to fully articulate a theory and method of psychoanalytic treatment based on Freud's second model of the mind* (Freud, 1923), specifically the newly defined role of the ego, further clarified in 1933 where Freud introduced the term "ego psychology" (p. 58) for the first time.[6] He also predicted the difficulty that analysts would have with this term:

> I must, however, let you know of my suspicion that this account of mine of *ego-psychology* will affect you differently from the introduction into the psychical underworld which preceded it. I cannot say with certainty why this should be so.
> (Freud, 1933, p. 58, italics added)

Freud was prescient in his prediction in that the theorists who had the most impact in Europe and Latin America after Freud (i.e., Bion, Klein, and Winnicott), almost never referenced Freud's second model of the mind, and for the most part, based their technique on Freud's first theory of anxiety. This is where he saw dammed-up libido as the cause of anxiety, so that deep interpretations of the unconscious were viewed as the only way to break the dam, freeing the libido.

In the United States, Ego Psychology was considered the basic theoretical perspective that most analysts accepted (Wallerstein, 2012), and while this was superficially true, there was no consistent method used that aligned with Freud's view of the ego. It is also not well known what Aisenstein (2014) pointed out: "I would like to remind the reader of the common roots of the 'American Ego Psychology' and what is presently called 'French Analysis'" (p. 1165).

An Outline of the Book

In the first two chapters of this book, I present, in condensed form, the theory and method that, I believe, is basic to a psychoanalytic cure. These are summary chapters where I try to capture the essence of what I've written about before, while offering the conclusions I've come to since writing *Creating a Psychoanalytic Mind* (2013). Chapters 3–12 include what I believe are new ways of understanding aspects of clinical psychoanalysis that augment what I've written in the first two chapters. Chapter 3 on self-analysis delves into the confusion about how this is achieved, and how I believe it can be achieved according to my model of the mind. Chapter 4 describes how Freud identified two kinds of transferences, but only one was prominent for some time. I've added a third transference based on what I've called "language action", which I believe is a part of every analysis. Chapter 5 discusses what I deem is essential in differentiating countertransference reactions to the patient's unconscious from the analyst's own conflicts. Chapter 6 discusses why transferences to people other than the analyst can be the most alive transference in the room. In Chapter 7, I present a new understanding of patients who are self-critical that adds to the literature on this topic. Silence is something that occurs in every analysis, but it is often treated as an epiphenomenon. Chapter 8 describes its importance and how it can be analyzed. I continue to explore the issue of resistance analysis, which was the first topic I wrote about in my 30-year journey of writing about the clinical implications of Freud's second model of the mind. I return to it in Chapter 9, where I differentiate two types of resistance analysis. The next three chapters are based on phenomena I've noticed with multiple patients that I don't believe have been portrayed in the way I do. In Chapter 10, I explore the concept of the importance of the analyst as a keeper of the patient's memories, while in Chapter 11 I use a scene from Martin Scorsese's movie *Taxi Driver*, to delve into the distinction between when the patient may be unconsciously communicating with the analyst, and when he may be attempting to repair a self-state. In the final chapter in this part, I present the case of a patient whose dreams were more like actions, designed to have an effect upon the analyst.

The next part of the book, for the most part, contains short chapters on our profession based on multiple observations over my half-century of involvement in psychoanalysis. However, there is one long chapter that explores "authority" in psychoanalytic institutes. I've appreciated the many articles on the problem with "authority" in psychoanalytic institutes, especially the work of Kernberg. I've approached the issue from a different perspective, mostly found in articles and books on higher education, where the problem of the post-modern approach to knowledge has been highlighted.

While writing this book, I've become aware of how old-fashioned it might appear to some. As I'm sure many have noticed, our meetings and journals have increasingly been dominated by panels and papers dealing with the crises facing the world. While I applaud this effort, I feel we've moved away from the many unresolved and crucial clinical issues that, I believe, are germane to clinical psychoanalysis. I hope that in these pages I've captured some of the issues that I see as essential to psychoanalytic treatment. I hope others will join me in this debate, and there will be more room for such discussions in our national and international meetings.[7]

Fred Busch
Chestnut Hill, MA
January 2024

Notes

1 One of the most important educational experiences in my post-doctoral training was a 2-year seminar where we read, page by page, Anna Freud's *Normality and Pathology in Childhood*, which had just been published.
2 A Freudian approach was the foundational perspective of many psychiatric departments at the time I trained.
3 At the time, it was thought there was a one-to-one correspondence between libidinal development and ego development, but Anna Freud's (1976) work dispelled this perspective.
4 One of my supervisors, the late Mayer Subrin, did help me see how staying closely attuned to the patient's associations led to interpretations that patients could understand, and often led to further associations which would be clarifying. He didn't present this way of working as based on any particular model of the mind, and I only realized later how well it fit within Freud's second model of the mind and the importance of the preconscious.
5 It appeared to me that Gray believed the analyst primarily needed to analyze resistances in order for patients to discover unconscious fantasies and conflicts. In my experience, analyzing resistances led to greater freedom in patients' preconscious associations that still needed to be clarified and interpreted by the analyst. Further, Gray didn't believe in the analyst's use of his countertransference in understanding patients.
6 Although I've written about this piece of analytic history many times, it is my impression that the distinction between Freud's first and second

models, and its clinical consequences, which I believe is crucial to analytic technique, are not so well understood by many analysts.

7   The reader will find several redundancies throughout the book. This is because there are certain ideas that are central to my perspective, and in order to fully articulate my perspective, I keep returning to them.

References

Aisenstein, M. (2014) Fred Busch's Creating a Psychoanalytical Mind: A Psychoanalytical Method and Theory. *Revue Française Psychoanalytic Technique* 78:1165–1172.

Aisenstein, M. and Smadja, C. (2010) Introduction to the Paper by Pierre Marty: The Narcissistic Difficulties Presented to the Observer by the Psychosomatic Problem. *International Journal of Psychoanalysis* 91:343–346.

Alexander, F. (1965) *Psychosomatic Medicine: Its Principles and Applications.* New York: Norton.

Brenner, C. (1982) *The Mind in Conflict.* Madison, CT: International Universities Press.

Busch, F. (1995) Do Actions Speak Louder Than Words? A Query Into an Enigma in Analytic Theory and Technique. *Journal of the American Psychoanalytic Association* 43:61–82.

Busch, F. (2006) A Shadow Concept. *International Journal of Psychoanalysis* 87:1471–1485.

Busch, F. (2009) 'Can You Push a Camel through the Eye of a Needle?' Reflections on how the Unconscious Speaks to us and its Clinical Implications. *International Journal of Psychoanalysis* 90:53–68.

Busch, F. (2013) *Creating a Psychoanalytic Mind.* London: Routledge.

Busch, F. (2015) Our Vital Profession. *International Journal of Psychoanalysis* 96:553–568.

Freud, Anna (1976) *Normality and Pathology in Children.* Madison, CT: International Universities Press.

Freud, S. (1923) The Ego and the Id. *S.E.* XIX.

Freud, S. (1933) The Dissection of the Psychical Personality. In the New Introductory Lectures On Psycho-Analysis. *S.E.* XXII: 57–80.

Green, A. (1974) Surface Analysis, Deep Analysis (The Role of the Preconscious in Psychoanalytical Technique). *International Review of Psychoanalysis* 1:415–423.

Green, A. (1975) The Analyst, Symbolization and Absence in the Analytic Setting (On Changes in Analytic Practice and Analytic Experience)—In Memory of D. W. Winnicott. *International Journal of Psychoanalysis* 56:1–22.

Rapaport, D., Gill, M. and Schafer, R. (1945) *Diagnostic Psychological Testing.* New York: Year-book Publisher.

Rapaport, D. (1951/1967) The Organization of Thought Processes. In Gill, M.M. (ed.), *The Collected Papers of David Rapaport.* New York: Basic Books.

Wallerstein, R.S. (2012) Will Psychoanalysis Fulfill its Promise? *International Journal of Psychoanalysis* 93:377–399.

Part I
Clinical Contributions

1   How Analysis Cures

The capacity of patients to tell and own their stories is central to their developing a sense of well-being from analysis. It is the basis of an exhilarating freedom from stories neurotically imposed by internal and external sources—the stories remembered but never integrated; the stories experienced but never formulated; the stories experienced and remembered only in the language of action; the stories of unconscious fantasy and defense; and the importance of all of these in every other story. Another more technical categorization might be that these are the stories of compromise formations and screen memories, stories enacted due to unstable structures or to thoughts represented in action form and stories based on implicit memories. In short, these are the stories of lives interrupted, manifested analytically in rigidly held, fearfully unknown, or incomplete stories.

But why is it important to unearth these stories and make them *representable*, which has always been the goal of psychoanalysis? How does this help our patients? The rest of this chapter will give my answer to these questions based upon what we've learned from psychoanalytic discoveries over the last 50 years. I will begin with a theoretical overview of the psychoanalytic landscape as a basis for my perspective and follow it with clinical examples.

Within my contemporary Freudian perspective, I would say the basis of the psychoanalytic curative process is *changing the inevitability of action into the possibility of reflection*. As Freud (1914) pointed out, patients come to our offices because they are driven to repeat, in action, the same behaviors over and over again. At the end of analysis, we hope patients can reflect upon what's propelling them towards certain thoughts, feelings, and behaviors, allowing them to make a choice before an action occurs. Pally and Olds (1998) liken it to the difference between a video recorder with and without memory storage. Without the capacity for memory storage, the individual is limited to respond to fleeting urges, while with it the individual has many images, thoughts, and feelings to compare and contrast with and reflect upon the immediate image. Our mind can process billions of pieces of information in less than one second, so the reflection I am referring to is the time of

DOI: 10.4324/9781032658704-3

an eye-blink, not a laborious, obsessional process. The reasons for my understanding the curative process this way follow.

There are two main factors that drive the patient to repeat, and repeat again, unconscious conflicts and fantasies, that limit his potential, and can derail any relationship. The first is the *insufficiency of representations*, and the second is the tendency toward action and what I call *"language action"*. I will first elaborate on building representations, and then discuss the importance of changing language action into thoughts and feelings. These are both an essential part of a psychoanalytic cure. In addition, I will discuss a particular type of knowledge (i.e., process knowledge) crucial to the patient's capacity to engage in self-analysis after the analysis has ended.

Building representations: A key factor in the curative process

It is my view that Freud's (1940) assessment of the *psychoanalytic curative* process still holds true: "its cure is a consequence of the analyst helping the weakened ego, giving it back *its mastery over lost provinces of his mental life*" (p. 175, italics added). Freud puts strengthening the ego at the center of the curative process.[1] But how does this strengthening of the ego occur? From the stand-point of theory and clinical evidence, the answer to the question of how the ego is strengthened seems simple ... *by building representations*. However, what this actually means is not simple. I will try to cover a vast territory by presenting a brief outline of what I think this concept, "building representations", means, and why it is central to my thinking. I will primarily present *my* understanding and a brief foray into the literature that presaged my perspective. I won't present a review of the surge of interest in the term "building representations" or my agreements and differences with those who have written about it. I am aware there are still many mysteries to be explored regarding this concept.

Why Building Representations is Important

One important way to think of why our patients come to us is that they suffer from insufficient representations. Without sufficient representations, the tendency is to move toward action, rather than having the capacity to consider alternatives. By action I don't mean a motoric process, but a way of thinking and feeling that *drives* a person in a particular direction. This is why, after multiple divorces, the next spouse turns out to be the same type of spouse, and after several moves to new jobs, every boss becomes the same boss. The more complex and unsaturated[2] representations are, the greater chance the patient has to reverse this process. It is in this way that the ego gains greater mastery over thoughts and feelings that the patient was buffeted by previous to psychoanalysis.

Since Freud's (1915) paper on the unconscious, building representations has always been the basic goal of psychoanalysis. However, what this meant only began to come into focus in the early 1950s, when psychoanalysts from two very different cultures began to articulate the significance of building representation, highlighting the importance of understanding the patient's *way of thinking*, rather than *only* focusing on the *content* of what patients think. Starting in the 1950s, some analysts began to write about the fact that for many patients, it was the lack of psychic representations that led to the repetitive nature of their problems. *This is one important way to think of the repetition compulsion ... as the failure of adequate representation.*

In the United States, the significance of representations can be found in the work of the brilliant David Rapaport, now largely forgotten. In a continuing refrain throughout his work, starting in the early 1940s, Rapaport emphasized the importance of thinking about *thoughts*. His major contribution was expressed this way:

> Though the understanding of *content* is sufficient for everyday communication and for many needs of diagnostic and therapeutic practice, it is insufficient for the understanding of personality and thought processes. *Consideration of contents will have to be supplemented and reinterpreted into formal characteristics of the thought process.*
>
> (1950, italics added)

At around the same time, French psychoanalysts began to highlight the importance of building *representations* to the curative process. Aisenstein and Smadja (2010) captured this perspective from one of the founders of the French Psychosomatic School, Pierre Marty (2010), when they pointed out the significant step Marty took in understanding psychosomatic patients: "it was not a question of looking for the *content* to give sense to the somatic symptoms but rather of observing the *inhibition or failures of psychic elaboration that proceed or accompany them*" (p. 343, italics added). Simply put, Marty saw the symptoms of psychosomatic patients as a result of a particular type of problem in thinking, or non-thinking ...that is, *the failure of representation*, rather than primarily the result of a physical enactment of an unconscious fantasy or conflict, which was central to the understanding of psychosomatic symptoms for many years and still is in some theoretical perspectives. The concept of representation, or lack thereof, has generally been central in French psychoanalysis. Green, in fact, sees the essential paradigm of psychoanalysis on the side of representation.[3]

In short, there has been a paradigm shift *across many psychoana-lytic cultures*, captured as the movement from only *lifting* repression to including a paradigm of *transformation*. That is, rather than *primarily* searching for buried memories, we attempt to transform the under-represented into ideas that are representable. For example, we attempt to build representations as a way of helping the patient *contain* previously threatening thoughts and feelings so that he can move toward deeper levels of meaning. What is represented can continue to build structure and enhance the ability to contain. This leads to what Green (1975) called "binding the inchoate" (p. 9) and containing it, thus giving a container to the patient's content and "content to his container" (p. 7).

To complicate matters, *representations are not there or not there, but are there in a variety of forms*. One can think of representations as having multiple dimensions, for example, from deeply unconscious to within the range of the preconscious, simple to complex; or degrees of saturation. In my view, building representations means attempting to make them more complex, closer to the preconscious, and less satu-rated (or more nuanced). In short, with a highly saturated, simple rep-resentation that is close to consciousness, we would attempt to make the representation more complex and less saturated. With a more com-plex representation that is unconscious, we would attempt to bring the representation to increasingly higher levels of preconsciousness.

Broadly speaking, then, there are ranges of representations we attempt to build. At a more primitive level, we attempt to build a simple representation from what is poorly represented and often expressed in the language of action, for example, helping a patient see they are *doing* something. At a more neurotic level, we help to build more complex representations by understanding the *meaning* in preconsciously formed associative links. In the first situation we are we are more like ethnographic researchers translating cave paintings into a written language, while in the second we are like a sophisticated translator who understands the music that goes with the words. In the first situation we are building a representation where previously there was primarily action. In the second we are building simple representa-tions into something more complex by adding links of meaning.

From Simple to Complex Representations

In this section, I will bring together data from nonpsychoanalytic sources that adds depth to the significance of building representa-tions as the most significant component of the curative process in psychoanalysis.

Westen and Gabbard (2002) explained to analysts the importance of neuronal pathways in distinguishing between the capacity for think-ing versus the tendency toward action. According to these authors, pieces of information are associatively connected to one another, so that activating one node (or unit of information) on a network spreads activation to other related nodes. Further, *knowledge lies in the connections among nodes in a network* (ibid., p. 74, italics in original), and *frequently used networks create attractor states* (ibid., p. 75, italics in original).

> The salience of traumatic memories keeps them at a high state of cognitive activation. This makes sense from an evolutionary perspective because events related to survival and reproduction should be readily and chronically activated. Once traumatized, we should remain vigilant toward situations that resemble the traumatic one. At the same time, however, the intense painful affect associated with traumatic memories activates inhibitory mechanisms defenses—aimed at keeping them out of awareness. This means they can never be worked through, and hence, paradoxically, the cognitive-affective network remains outside awareness even while being readily triggered.
>
> (ibid., p. 84)

Evidence from the field of neuroplasticity supports this idea. This field revolves around the idea that it is the ability of neural networks *in the* brain to have the capacity *to change through growth and reorganization*. It is when the brain is rewired to function in some way that differs from how it previously functioned. What is pertinent for psychoanalysis is *the capacity for neuronal pathways* to *make new connections*. Neuroplasticity was once thought by neuroscientists to be manifest only during childhood, but research from the 1960s on showed that many aspects of the brain can be altered (or are "plastic") even through adulthood. Structural plasticity is often understood as the brain's ability to change its neuronal connections. *I suggest that in psychoanalysis, building representations can increase the number of neuronal networks, thus changing what was at a high level of activation into thoughts that can be thought.*[4]

I find it remarkable that Freud (1913, 1918) was describing the importance of plasticity at a much earlier time. "The extraordinary diversity of the psychical constellations concerned, the *plasticity* of all mental processes and the wealth of determining factors oppose any mechanization of the technique" (1913, p. 123).

To repeat, by building complex representations, *we change the inevitability of action to the possibility of reflection.* As one patient described it:

> I was thinking about all the things I had to do, making lists, fretting about how I could get it all done ... but as soon as I was able to

think "I feel under a lot of pressure to *do something*", my tendency to fill up my world with doing to avoid thinking came back to me, and the pressure disappeared.

Repeating in Action

As I mentioned earlier, moving from action to thinking and feeling is, in my mind, an essential element in the curative process. Here is how my understanding evolved.

Throughout my analytic training, and afterwards, I noticed a pattern that seemed consistent amongst the patients I saw. That is, the patient would be talking, and the shape of something important would emerge that seemed to open a window into the conflicts or narcissistic issues that brought him[5] to psychoanalysis. However, at a certain point, he would still be talking, but what he said shed little light on what he'd just been talking about. Further, I became aware of feelings I was having that I couldn't connect to anything the patient was saying with words.

It was at a time in my Institute when we were taught that the kind of feelings I was having were considered a countertransference and necessitated further analysis. Gallahorn (1993) captured the atmosphere where I trained in the following ways:

> Within our traditional institute which emphasizes an ego psychological approach to clinical work, the candidates are aware of countertransference in themselves but experience it *primarily* as something bad which must be overcome rather than understood. It is seen by the candidates as evidence of their imperfection.
>
> (p. 322)[6]

Thus, I didn't bring my countertransference feelings into supervision but continued to be intrigued by the phenomenon. Sometime later I remembered reading Freud's (1914) article "Remembering, Repeating and Working Through", and I re-read it. There I found a passage that clearly seemed important when I first read it, as it was heavily underlined. Freud wrote:

> There are some cases which behave like those under the hypnotic technique up to a point and only later cease to do so; but others behave differently from the beginning. If we confine ourselves to this second type in order to bring out the difference, we may say that the patient does not *remember* anything of what he has forgotten and repressed but *acts* it out. He reproduces it not as a memory but as an action; he *repeats* it, without, of course, knowing that he

is repeating it. For instance, the patient does not say that he remembers that he used to be defiant and critical towards his parents' authority; instead, he behaves in that way to the doctor.

He does not remember how he came to a helpless and hopeless deadlock in his infantile sexual researches but he produces a mass of confused dreams and associations, complains that he cannot succeed in anything and asserts that he is fated never to carry through what he undertakes. He does not remember having been intensely ashamed of certain sexual activities and afraid of their being found out; but he makes it clear that he is ashamed of the treatment on which he is now embarked and tries to keep it secret from everybody.

(ibid., p. 150)

Later in this brief paper Freud goes on to say, "As long as the patient is in the treatment, he cannot escape from this compulsion to repeat; and in the end we understand that this is his way of remembering" (ibid., p. 150).

Language Action

In his 1914 paper, Freud described this phenomenon of repetitions in *action* but didn't give any reasons as to why this action occurs. Why would it be that the closer one comes to expressions of the unconscious in psychoanalysis, it would be expressed in the language of action? I have offered one hypothesis, which is that *thought is under the domination of action for a much longer period of time than has generally been recognized in psychoanalysis.* The reason for this "action" type of thinking has to do, in part, with the way thought processes develop. One of the major characteristics of all intelligence is that it is a matter of action. As Basch (1981) demonstrated, imaging is not the foundation for thought; action encoded in sensori-motor schema is that foundation. The main distinction between different stages of intellectual development is the degree to which actions become internalized and behavior is based upon representations rather than a motoric underpinning. It is important to note that the process of internalization is a very lengthy one. It is not until a child is around age 7 that one can talk of his having an integrated cognitive system with which he can organize the world relatively free from action referents.[8] Before that time, the child's thinking is heavily influenced by its motoric underpinnings. For example, a 5-year-old can successfully walk to school and negotiate a number of school corridors to find his kindergarten class, but he is unable to reproduce this in representational form, as his thinking is of a "doing" type. The younger the child, the more his thinking will be dominated by action. For children capable of higher-level function-ing, conflict and regression will heighten the tendency toward thinking based on action.

Thus, what has not been sufficiently emphasized is that actions become increasingly woven into the fabric of the psychoanalytic process, in part, because of the long period of time the child's thinking remains under the influence of action determinants. Central conflicts and the adaptations to them are first experienced, organized, and worked out at an *action* level. Whatever the danger, the original defensive adapta-tions and compromise formations were undertaken in action terms, and thus may remain unavailable to higher-level ego functioning or remain in waiting as regressive flash points. *Up until the oedipal phase and its crucial importance in shaping psychic development, action tendencies remain as a primary mode of the child's thought processes.*

So, what is earliest and most primitive in the unconscious is stored in action-thoughts. Thus, the closer we come to what is unconscious, the more likely patients will express themselves via action. The deeper we go into the unconscious, *and it is useful to think of gradients in the unconscious,* the more thought is equated with action. What is most unconscious is always enacted. Think of our most disturbed patients where, in areas of their disturbance, thoughts are closer to reflex actions. As Loewald (1971, 1975) noted, the deeper one goes in psy-choanalysis, the greater likelihood the patient will express themselves in the language of action.

Two Types of Knowledge

My basic premise is that there is a need to create two types of knowl-edge in psychoanalysis.[7] *State* knowledge is what psychoanalysts are most familiar with. That is, we help make representations more complex by interpreting the multiple ways a patient's search for a better mother shows itself in his life and interferes with his goals, along with the factors that led him to this position. The patient ends analysis *knowing* that he has this problem and the multiple ways it is expressed, along with the specific interaction of the drives with exter-nal circumstances that led to this pattern. In short, the way most of us have been taught to practice in the international community is that knowledge of the unconscious is what patients most urgently need to know. Our basic theory suggests that the more of these unconscious elements we can bring into awareness, the less likely the pull of their manifestations in action will occur. There is, of course, a great deal of merit in this perspective. However, there is another perspective to be considered, which is that *the process of knowing is as important as what is known.* It is my underlying thesis in *creating a psycho-analytic mind* (Busch, 2013) that what is accomplished in a relatively successful psychoanalysis is *a way of knowing*, and not simply knowing. My experience in doing second analyses is that patients often come in knowing a lot, but they *don't know how to know*. They are stuck in knowing what they learned from their analyst in a previous treatment and can't continue to grow and develop when the exigencies of life arouse variations of previous anxieties. It can lead to a belief in a kind of knowing we might call formulaic intuition. Its expression can be seen in patients who, when hearing a surprising association, say something like, "Oh, that must be my critical father (mother, sister, brother, etc.) emerging", or "That must be my fractured self", or "my homosexual side". These are "insights" that stop thinking rather than stimulate it. They can become part of a self-deceptive personal narrative to protect from unconscious fears and/or enacted wishes.

Process knowledge comes, in part, from analyzing the process of knowing. It requires a different form of attention that focuses on analyzing the patient's way of analyzing, the resistances to analyzing, and the analyst's way of bringing what he knows. It leads a patient into a different psychological state that I call a *psychoanalytic mind. This is where the analysand has a different relationship to his thoughts and feelings than previously, seeing them as psychological events that can be observed, thought about, and played with.*

In the midst of conflict, patients often think of their thoughts primarily as realities. They think, but they cannot think about their thinking. At these times, a man describing an argument with his wife is not wondering why these thoughts may be on his mind. He can't observe his thoughts as thoughts, let alone reflect or play with them. Over time, certain methods of working (to be discussed in the next chapter) along with a focus on the process lead to a change in the analysand's capacity to become the kind of thinker capable of a self-analytic capacity. It is this method that more often leads to self-analysis rather than an identification with the analyst's functioning, which has been the primary way the development of self-analysis has been hypothesized. In short, process knowledge works differently than state knowledge. Process knowledge leads to an appreciation of the methods necessary to obtain state knowledge. Process knowledge is not silent. It is the result of active, but not directed, mental activity. It often has the quality of a daydream, but unlike a daydream, where the dreamer luxuriates in his thoughts, process thinking includes the capacity for an observing ego and the ability to play with thoughts for self-knowledge.

In short, at the heart of *process knowledge is the capacity to think of one's thoughts as mental events.* This seemingly simple capacity is a hard-won accomplishment for all patients in analysis. However, the benefits are enormous, as it potentially allows the patient to step back and reflect rather than act.

Green (2005) captured the idea of *process knowledge* in the following statement: "the aim of an interpretation is not to produce insight directly but to facilitate the psychic functioning that is likely to help insight" (p. 5).

Creating Process Knowledge

George was a meek 19-year-old who came to analysis because of the difficulty he had going off to college. He'd been accepted at a prestigious university the previous year but had been unable to start the semester because of a series of vague maladies, where no medical cause could be found. He knew he was anxious and panicky about leaving home but kept this to himself to avoid what he felt would be his father's condemnation and his mother's pity. After two years of analysis, George felt he was ready to start college. He'd arranged with a friend who went to the same school to drive him to college to begin his freshman year. When he told his mother this, she became angry and then started crying. First, she berated him because the guy he was driving with was a "flake". He stood up for his friend by reminding his mother that she hadn't been around him since high school, that he matured a lot since then, and in fact had received some prestigious academic awards. However, nothing could convince his mother at this time, and she went to her bedroom, where George could hear her muffled sobbing. Later in the day she came back to George and apologized to him. She said she realized she was very upset about his leaving, and that she wanted to drive him to college so she could be with him as long as she could. At some point she realized this was selfish on her part, and it didn't fit with what he needed. (In fact, at George's suggestion, his mother went into analysis, and had become less narcissistic.) Shortly after his mother apologized, George retreated to a meek, ineffective way of being, and reassured his mother he'd be home on many weekends, and he became confused about how he'd get home, unconsciously inviting his mother to step in and inform him of the necessary steps he needed to take to return home. At this point I said:

> After asserting yourself with your mother about your plans, she was initially upset but then she was able to apologize to you for how she reacted. At that point it seemed to me you felt uneasy about this, retreated, and became again the meek boy who needed his mother to show him what to do.

In this interpretation of a regressive defense, I am attempting to do a number of things to bring about process knowledge:

1. To bring to George's attention the sequence of his association, indicating it is *what comes to his mind* that is the basis of understanding. As indicated previously (Busch, 2009, 2013), throughout much of an analysis a patient is not able to follow their own associations. It is only later in analysis that a patient is able to step back from following his associations, and reflect upon them. Therefore, I try to capture the thread of his associations, and play them back to him before suggesting any meaning. In this way the analyst briefly becomes an auxiliary ego. We can only learn the "meaning" from the patient's further associations. If the patient cannot associate, it likely means he wasn't ready for this interpretation.

2. In my interpretation, I'm using what Steiner (1994) called an "analyst-centered" method of interpretation. This is where the analyst interprets based upon his impressions or thoughts, rather than giving what I call "you are" interpretations (e.g., "you're angry right now"). In this way, we can potentially lessen the effects of superego self-condemnations. We do this by also making our interventions more tentative.

3. I find many interpretations analysts make come from their own mind, based upon whatever theoretical position they hold. It is different than trying to talk *with* patients about what they're able to tell us, via their associations. Here is an example of what I mean from a respected psychoanalyst working from a different theoretical perspective. *At issue here is from what position the analyst interprets and helps or hinders the patient's ability to understand how to use his own mind.*

Brown (2015) tells us that in the third year of treatment, the patient suddenly announces he is terminating the treatment at the end of the session and does so. My thoughts are in italics:

Mr. R's sudden decisions to immediately end the analysis, though clearly related to fears of dependency and homoerotic anxieties, occurred without any apparent warning: he simply and calmly said he was not returning and thanked me for my help. The manner in which he abruptly ended our work understandably left me feeling blindsided, weak, and helpless. As I reflected on Mr. R's mode of ending, it seemed clear that his feelings of "gayness" and dependency had been projected into me and had now become my burden with which to struggle, leaving me feeling weakened and impotent.

(pp. 852–853)

When the patient returned to treatment Brown puts his own feelings back into the patient when he says, "After his return, I brought up his leaving suddenly as a means by which he got rid of feeling weak and gay, and instead sought to evoke those emotions in me—i.e., 'giving' them to me as my problem to handle" (pp. 852–853). The patient superficially agreed with this intervention, but it seemed to have no effect upon him, according to Brown. So rather than listening to what the patient has to say about his abruptly leaving the analysis and then coming back, Brown pre-emptively interprets from his own theory of what is occurring.

Here the model the analyst is working within is that it is knowledge gained by the analyst's understanding of his countertransference that is most important. This model necessitates the patient's identification with the analyst, rather than process knowledge, as the way towards self-analysis. (See Chapter 6 for another elaboration of dealing with countertransference feelings.)

What About … ?

Inevitably, when I present my perspective on the curative process, someone will ask, "What about … " and then will complete the question by mentioning the significance of factors outlined by other perspectives. While I generally agree with the additional factor the questioner is asking about, I follow this by reiterating a position I've taken previously, which is, while I believe there are many factors that play a role in the good-enough analysis, I see them as necessary but not sufficient to qualify as the main agents of change in analysis. For example, I think it is important to try and create an atmosphere of safety and being non-judgmental in analytic sessions, but this by itself does not make an analysis. It is a helpful addition, but not the essence of a psychoanalytic cure. Of course, it is important to remember that whatever our intentions may be, it doesn't mean this is how the patient will experience the situation, which is determined by their unconscious fantasies, conflicts, and defenses.

Notes

1 Feldman (2007), writing from a different theoretical position also points to "the *functions* of the interpretation in promoting the analytic process by strengthening the ego," (p. 613).
2 Saturated and unsaturated representations have to do with the degree that an unconscious representation is filled with ideas and feelings that bring the person to a single conclusion. Thus, an unsaturated representation would be characterized by multiple ideas about a particular object, while a saturated representation would lead a person to a singular view of the object.

3 It's my impression that, according to Bronstein, what differentiates a Kleinian view from the Paris school is that Kleinians address psychosomatic illness by exploring the unconscious phantasies and psychic conflicts that underlie psychosomatic symptoms as well as the different defense mechanisms.

4 I am using "thoughts" here as short-hand version of "thoughts and feelings".

5 In the interest of readability the use of the masculine and feminine pronouns will be dispensed with. All references to persons apply equally to both genders.

6 Gallahorn was describing the atmosphere in his Institute. Gallahorn and I were in different Institutes, but the attitudes towards countertransference feelings were similar.

7 For a fuller explanation of these two types of knowledge, see Busch, 2013, Chapter 2.

References

Aisenstein, M. ānd Smadja, C. (2010) Introduction to the Paper by Pierre Marty: The Narcissistic Difficulties Presented to the Observer by the Psychosomatic Problem. *International Journal of Psychoanalysis* 91:343–346.

Basch, M. F. (1981) Psychoanalytic Interpretation and Cognitive Transformation. *International Journal of Psychoanalysis* 62:151-175.

Brown, L.J. (2015) Ruptures in the Analytic Setting and Disturbances in the Transformational Field of Dreams. *Psychoanalytic Quarterly* 84(4):841–865.

Busch, F. (2009) 'Can You Push a Camel Through the Eye of a Needle?' Reflections on How the Unconscious Speaks to us and its Clinical Implications. *International Journal of Psychoanalysis* 90:53–-56.

Busch, F. (2013) *Creating a Psychoanalytic Mind*. London: Routledge.

Busch, F. (2015) Our Vital Profession. *International Journal of Psychoanalysis* 96:553–568.

Feldman, M. (2007) The Illumination of History. *International Journal of Psychoanalysis* 88:609–625.

Freud, S. (1913) On Beginning the Treatment (Further Recommendations on the Technique of Psycho-Analysis I). *S.E.* 12:121–144.

Freud, S (1914) Remembering, Repeating and Working-Through. *S.E.* 12:145–156.

Freud, S. (1915) The Unconscious. *S.E.* 14:159–215.

Freud, S. (1918) From the History of an Infantile Neurosis. *S.E.* 17:1–124.

Freud, S. (1940) An Outline of Psycho-Analysis. *International Journal of Psychoanalysis* 21:27–84.

Gallahorn, G.E. (1993) George E. Gallahorn. *Journal of Clinical Psychoanalysis* 2:321–323.

Green, A. (1975) The Analyst, Symbolization and Absence in the Analytic Setting (On Changes in Analytic Practice and Analytic Experience)—In Memory of D. W. Winnicott. *International Journal of Psychoanalysis* 56:1–22.

Green, A. (2005) The Illusion of Common Ground and Mythical Pluralism. *International Journal of Psychoanalysis* 86:627–632.

Loewald, H. (1971) Some Comments on Repetition and Repetition Compulsion. *International Journal of Psychoanalysis* 52:59-66.

Loewald, H. (1975). Psychoanalysis as an Art and the Fantasy Character of the Psychoanalytic Situation. *Journal of the American Psychoanalytic Association*, 23(2):277-299.

Marty, P. (2010) The Narcissistic Difficulties Presented to the Observer by the Psychosomatic Problem. *International Journal of Psychoanalysis* 91:347–360.

Pally, R. and Olds, D. (1998) Consciousness: A Neuroscience Perspective. *International Journal of Psychoanalysis* 79:971–989.

Rapaport, D. (1950) On the Psycho-Analytic Theory of Thinking. *International Journal of Psychoanalysis* 31:161–170.

Steiner, J. (1994) Patient-Centered and Analyst-Centered Interpretations: Some Implications of Containment and Countertransference. *Psychoanalytic Inquiry* 14:406–422.

Westen, D. and Gabbard, G. O. (2002) Developments in Cognitive Neuroscience: I. Conflict, Compromise, and Connectionism. *Journal of the American Psychoanalytic Association* 50:53–98.

2 Methods of Interpretation

While the main goal of interpreting is to build representations, there are *ways of building representations* that aid the patient in becoming his own analyst, and ways that lead the patient to remain dependent on what they learned from their analyst. I have consistently noticed that when I see patients in a second analysis, they search for answers to their problems in previous interpretations from their analyst, which interferes with the freedom to follow their own thoughts wherever they may lead, and thus find new insights.

I would suggest the main goal of any intervention during psychoanalysis is that it should be based upon *what the patient has communicated, and is emotionally meaningful, and cognitively understandable.* We want the patient to feel touched by what we say, and potentially understand how we came to make our interventions. However, as soon as I use the phrase, "what the patient has communicated" a thicket of conflicting ideas come to mind that need further elaboration. This is especially the case when it comes to the idea that the analyst can understand something about the patient's unconscious via countertransference and reverie. For many analysts, the patient's associations have moved far into the background as the most important source of information for what is *interpretable.* In my theory of therapeutic action, it is the patient's use of free association that is the most important source of information that is usable for interpretation. This is because patients' associations are most often what is preconsciously available until the inevitable resistances come to the fore. Working with what is preconsciously available to the patient, as well as analyzing the defenses against certain content emerging into awareness is, in my understanding, the best way to interpret without arousing unbearable anxiety. In working slowly, we help the patient move towards understanding his unconscious.[1]

There are, of course, other ways patients communicate what is going on in their minds. Earlier, I pointed to language action as one-way patients communicate with their analyst. This is when patients' words are meant to *do* things to or with the analyst. Language action is not as close to preconscious awareness as most verbal associations are, and it generally takes longer for the analyst to understand what

DOI: 10.4324/9781032658704-4

is happening. Eventually this way of communicating serves as a resistance and needs to be interpreted. We start by detailing for the patient how the language action is shown. For example, in the case of a patient who talks so fast the analyst can't follow her thoughts, the analyst doesn't have the luxury of musing on the patient's verbalizations or have much space to say anything to the patient. At a certain point, I might interrupt the patient and say, "Have you noticed you talk very fast. At times I find it difficult to follow you or have the space to say anything." I would leave this as an unsaturated clarification and wait to see the patient's reaction to understand how to proceed.

From a different perspective, I find too many interventions I hear analysts make are more "moi interpretations", that is, coming from the analyst's own mind based upon his theory, rather than following what the patient can communicate. Here is an example of an interpretation that I understand as a "moi interpretation". Within the analyst's theory, I have no doubt he sees his interpretation as the correct one, and others of the same persuasion would agree with him.

Michael Feldman (2007), who always impresses me as one of the most creative post-Kleinians, reports that a patient was hostile and provocative in the session, announcing that she had binged on food and alcohol the previous weekend. Hearing this, Feldman felt frustration, anger, and hopelessness. The patient mentioned in passing that she hadn't been short-listed for a job she had applied for. Using his countertransference reaction as a guide to a projective identification, Feldman takes up how disturbing this had been for her and suggests that *it resonated with her feeling she didn't have a place with the analyst*. He then reports saying, "I thought these experiences contributed to the hostile dismissive way in which I was now being treated, as the person who was unsuited for the particular job".

Miss B was silent for a while, and then spoke in a moving way about feeling that a door had been closed on her. She also mentioned how complicated and painful it had been for her to visit her sister and her new baby. On the following day (the Friday before the long weekend), she arrived late, and told me that she was feeling very ill. It had been a great struggle to get up and to come, and she really shouldn't have. She said she had been "drinking mercilessly" the night before—she "drank and drank and drank". She stayed for about half the session, and then said she felt too unwell, and needed to go home (p. 617).

After Feldman's interpretation, the patient's first reaction is silence, which Feldman doesn't analyze (See Chapter 8 for a discussion of patients' silences). The patient then didn't react to Feldman's interpretation of the transference, but instead elaborated on how she felt "a door was being closed". Feldman, like many analysts who tend to seek out the transference, assumed the patient's reactions (i.e., binging on food and alcohol) were to the upcoming long weekend and being away from the analyst, rather than the possibility of the patient needing to do these things in order to protect a self-state or many other possibilities (see Chapter 9 for an elaboration of this point). It is my impression that in Feldman's example, he doesn't focus on what I would see as crucial: the *defense* against the awareness of the feelings of disappointment over not being short-listed, leading to her drinking over the weekend. See Chapter 6 on the external transference). *Left unexplored is why the patient was unable to be aware of how much she was affected by this news, but instead had to blunt her feelings with excessive drinking and binging.* Instead, it is interpreted directly as part of an unconscious transference reaction. If the patient had to *drown out any feelings of disappointment over the weekend*, why would we assume that she could accept the analyst telling her this was what she was feeling, let alone that she was enacting this with the analyst, where now he is the unacceptable one? It is indeed an interpretation at the deepest level of anxiety at the moment. As one can see in the next session the patient continues to need to drown her feelings after Feldman's intervention. As Schafer (1994) noted, Kleinians have not adequately developed a position on matters of importance in standard Freudian structural and functional theory (e.g., defense analysis).

In general, I find analysts looking for the transference rather than finding it. We tend to be more eager to bring the transference into the room, rather than letting it be in the room. We seem to believe that unless we are addressing the transference, we aren't doing real analytic work. Green (1974) noted one problem in strictly focusing on the transference. While he believes the transference is the driving force in analysis, he reminds us that analysis conducted primarily around the transference puts undue pressure on the patient. "The analysis takes on an aspect of persecution even if these interpretations are designed to help the patient understand what is happening within him" (ibid, p. 416).

It is my impression that recent theoretical developments have led to psychoanalysts abandoning the use of free association as the primary method of understanding the patient. However, as early as 1931 Freud was concerned that psychoanalysts were drifting away from the use of free association. In a letter to Stephen Zweig, he wrote, "You hardly mention the technique of free association, considered by many people the most important contribution made by psychoanalysis, the methodological key to its results" (p. 403).

What do I mean by using the patient's free associations as the basis for interpreting? I will present detailed examples throughout the book but let me present a brief vignette to give you an idea of what I'm describing.

Free Association and Creating Process Knowledge

Sylvia, age 45, was a successful academic who came to analysis at her husband's urging. At various times during their marriage, she was convinced he was having an affair even though she had no concrete evidence she could point to. Over time, a number of other issues arose, most importantly her competitive relationship with men, which helped her gain academic prizes and admiration from younger female academics but seemed to frequently lead to arguments with her male colleagues. One day when she was talking about her childhood, she wondered if she ever told me that her bedroom was next to her parents' bedroom, and when she was younger, she would hear these noises like her parents were fighting. However, after such nights, the next morning at breakfast her parents seemed especially happy. When she was a teenager, and had her first experience of intercourse, she heard the noises her partner and she were making, and in a flash of insight, she figured out these noises she heard from her parents' bedroom came from her parents having sex. She remembered that shortly after this recognition she became very angry with her parents, especially her father. She was puzzled by this because up until that time she was closest to her father. Yet, she remained estranged from her father for many years.

In one session she reported the following. She was working in her study at home one evening, when she heard her husband talking on the phone in his study, which was right next to hers. It sounded to her like her husband was excitedly talking to this person, and alternately like he was whispering. She immediately thought he was talking to a lover. She tried to put this out of her mind but couldn't. With some shame, after her husband went to sleep, she went to his study to see who he was speaking to. When she looked at his phone, she saw that the call she heard came from his best friend Howard. She briefly felt relieved, but then "realized" they could have been talking about an affair her husband was having, and she became angry at him.

FB: As I've mentioned before I have no way of knowing if your husband is having an affair, but if we follow your thoughts, when you hear these sounds from the room next to you, you're convinced it is the sound of your husband talking to a lover. When you check his phone and see it was Howard, you're momentarily relieved, but then return to the possibility they could have been talking about your husband's lover. At this point it was my impression that you felt propelled to believe your husband was having an affair.

Sylvia: It's true, when you replay what I just said it does seem like I need to believe this for some reason. But why? I can hear you saying, "that's a good question". After a brief pause, Sylvia said, "A conversation I had with my mother came to mind. She was her usual self, distant and distracted. I don't know why I keep hoping she's going to be any different. Remember I told you about Joan, a new hire in our Department that I offered to mentor. But it's clear she wants to get in with the big guys, and they will be glad to accept this attractive, bright 25-year-old. I felt angry, not at Joan, but these 'Big. Guys' who want to claim her.

FB: When you wonder why you may need to believe your husband is having an affair, your thoughts go to the frustrating call with your mother, which seemed to mirror your experience of her growing up. While you were talking about hearing your husband in the next room, I was reminded of another time you heard noises from the next room and believed, for some time, your father was beating up your mother before realizing they were having sex and blamed him for your mother's unavailability to you.

Sylvia: Interesting! I can see how you came to that. Part of me is appreciative that you were able to make that connection, and another part is annoyed that you saw it first.

FB: So even though you can appreciate what I said, it seems to lead you to feel competitive with me, which is what seems to happen sometimes with men.

In this vignette, one can see that by listening to Sylvia's associations and bringing them to her attention before bringing my understanding, I convey that it is by listening to her thoughts we can understand what is most important. It is a way of introducing the importance of process knowledge.

Of course, with some patients we have to pay attention to the music accompanying their words (i.e., the way they present thoughts, rather than the thoughts themselves). Ogden (2007) provides an excellent example of what I'm describing, although this is not his emphasis. A patient in her second year of analysis had lost all hope that her analyst could be of any help to her. Most of what Ogden describes then is the analytic *process* and what the patient is *doing*. "She spoke spasmodically, blurting out clumps of words, as if trying to get as many words as she could into each breath of air" (p. 578). "She barely paused after I spoke before continuing the line of thought that I had momentarily interrupted" (p. 578). The patient flooded "the sessions with clump after clump of words" (p. 578). Ogden's interpretation is of this *process not the content*. He next tells us that over several months the patient's speech became less pressured. I bring this as an example of how the intuitive clinician senses the need to work with the music that accompanies the words, not just the words themselves.

Instead of following the twists and turns of a patient's associations as the basic data of analysis, I find analysts

- listen for a *moment* where there is some content the analyst you believes explains something, and only focuses on this one moment rather than the flow of associations.

- Or they get a sense of the overall gestalt of what the patient is *unconsciously* expressing and use this as the core of an interpretation.
- Or they listen to what is stirred up in them in the form of *feelings or a reverie* that is used as the basis of an interpretation.
- Or they listen primarily to see what can be understood in the transference.

While I believe there are times when using all of these types of data can be important, as an overall approach it leads to a view of analysis as the *analyst as expert*, and it is only through his special knowledge that the patient can gain insight. When I hear talented psychoanalysts present clinical material, I often find they're excellent at building *state* knowledge, but miss producing *process* knowledge. That is, they help patients *know* something about their conflicts, fantasies, defenses, etc., but they don't help patients *know how to know*...an essential element in creating a psychoanalytic mind. Using a patient's associations as a basis for helping her appreciate what is going on in her mind is, I believe, indispensable in creating a psychoanalytic mind. Thus, a key element in interpreting in a manner that builds toward creating a psychoanalytic mind is *how we communicate our understanding* to a patient, not just *what* we communicate. Crucial, also, is to convey to a patient that we understand them, primarily, *by listening to what is coming to her mind*. What we don't want the analyst to consistently do is to communicate that it is *only* through her empathy, knowledge, or warmth that analysis progresses. If this does occur, it makes it difficult for the patient to find her own mind and engage in self-analysis based upon the necessity of listening to her own mind. Much of the literature on self-analysis describes it as a result of an identification with the analyst's functioning. While self-analysis may be a by-product of good analytic work, *I think it is also a result of the way the analyst analyzes.* Schacter (1992), amongst many others, has suggested the importance of the capacity for self-analysis in the termination phase. However, he, like many, sees self-analysis as developing *via identifying with the analyst's analyzing function.* In contrast, I believe that *by analyzing in a particular fashion we create the conditions for the patient's relationship to his own mind that allows self-analysis to take place.*

Before delving further into my method of interpreting, it seems important to say a few words about my view of free association. My basic assumption in using the psychoanalytic method is that most of what we need to know can be found in the patient's use of *the method of free association*. In the patient's use of the method of free association, we can see how unknown thoughts guide her, inhibit her, and destroy her. We can also come to understand the process by which patients guide, inhibit, and destroy their thoughts. Thus, we can learn how effective our methods are (or are not) in increasing the freedom of mind to say or not to say thoughts that are coming to mind. Sometimes thoughts are told in words, sometimes in the absence of words. Sometimes they are more like actions, designed to have us love, hate, believe, or suspect the patient (Busch, 2013, pp. 46–56). All of this comes in an order and sequence we cannot ask about because it follows the individual fabric of the patient's preconscious or unconscious mind at the moment.

I would suggest then, *in one form or another*, everything that happens in an analytic session is a free association. An evasion is never *just an evasion,* what seems unrelated is *never unrelated,* what seems boring is never *just boring.* While an obsessional patient may drone on about a moment in his history that he's gone over before, he is *communicating* something, for example, a resistance to something in the present, an attempt to help us understand something in a different way, a transference reaction to some exciting thought, an attempt to make the analyst feel something, etc. In broad-brush strokes, the analysand is always *communicating* something or *doing* something. Free association is not something the patient is supposed to do, but *what they are doing.* Kris (1982) stated it most succinctly when he said: "Psychoanalysis does not create free association in the treatment setting. It merely provides an alteration in the condition of ordinary association. … It replaces silent soliloquy with spoken words" (p. 14).

It is how the analyst uses the patient's associations that differentiates whether we are creating *process* knowledge or *state* knowledge. Below are two examples of the analyst interpreting in a way that leads to these different forms of knowledge. In the first example there is a vignette that demonstrates what I believe is a typical way many analysts interpret to patients, that is, based upon the analyst's understanding, she tells the analysand *what he's thinking*, which leads *to state* knowledge. I will have no question about the *content* of the analyst's interpretation, only the *form*.

Anonymous

The example is from the analyst at work series in the *International Journal of Psychoanalysis* (Anonymous, 2022). It revolves around the second session where the analysand comes to analysis in person, after a long time working by phone because of Covid. There also seems to have been some interruption in having regular appointments for reasons that aren't explained. After the analysand has a number of associations about his state of mind where he vacillates between worrying about himself and feeling he is doing well. The analyst then makes her first interpretation.

Analyst: Much is going on at the moment. In the last few weeks, you did not have access to the regularity and stability of your

sessions. Then we moved back to the office, which is also creating a sense of imbalance, a little tremor. And all this is in the
context of ending our work at some point in the foreseeable
future. You seem to want me to know that you need to hold on
to something familiar and stable in any way you can, like your
analysis, while also remembering you did attain stability after
having these tremors in the past.

Patient: Why are those aspects showing? Why am I asking you why
I do such and such again. I remember talking about whether
asking questions were helpful or important. At the time I felt
dismissed. Then I thought if I bring these aspects from earlier
times, and I know they stabilize, because you help me. I know
you are still the same person you were then, and what I'm telling
you are thoughts and vestiges from the past. I am now picturing
the cats bringing in worms to the kitchen and I throw them out.
They bring them back, even snakes. I throw them out again or
they bring the toy worm to play catch. I want to make sure that
you will handle what I bring to you the same way you did before
or am I trying to analyze myself here.

Analyst: You are making sure that I hear that you are worried about
beginning office sessions as well as the end of analysis, worried
about not having your internal voice guiding you. That when
you stop seeing me, be in my presence, you will lose my voice.

*As one can see, in her first interpretation, the analyst interprets eve-
rything the patient's is saying around issues of separation from the
analyst, without helping the patient understand how she came to
this conclusion. How does the patient respond? The first statement
I noticed was the patient wondering, "Why am I asking you why I
do such and such again?" Here I wondered whether the analysand
asks for the analyst's understanding because this is the analyst's established method, that is, the patient associates and the analyst interprets
according to her understanding. He then mentions that he asked this
question before, that is, 'why am I asking you for answers?', and felt
dismissed, which the analyst doesn't explore. He then likens the analytic process to what happens with his cat. The cat brings in what to the
cat are little treasures but are thrown out. I can see how the analysand
might experience the analysis in this way. In fact, this is what seemed
to happen in the analyst's second interpretation. What to me seem like
important transference associations (i.e., dismissed questions and the
cat metaphor) don't appear in the analyst's interpretation. Instead,
the analyst interprets, in what seems to me a global fashion, the same
theme of separation touched on in the first interpretation.*

*Here's an interpretation I might make that brings in the transfer-
ence question the patient seems able to express in a preconscious form*

as the treatment is drawing to a close..."how can he understand the thoughts that are coming to his mind" ?

> My interpretation: When you wonder why you're asking me for answers, I think you're bringing up an important question that you felt I've dismissed...and maybe I have. I wonder if your thoughts about the cat, and the things it brings in from outside, may be how you've experienced how I deal with your thoughts...not appreciating or valuing them as important, but rather tossing them out like something unwanted, and replaced by my own thoughts.

While there are certain topics in this interpretation that need to be elaborated further, and I will, for now I want to stay with my main point of interpreting in a way that builds a psychoanalytic mind. As the reader can see, I bring in the sequence of the patient's thoughts as a way of explaining why I'm making the interpretation. In this way I'm showing that, if we listen to your thoughts, you'll be able to understand what's upsetting you. This becomes the framework for self-analysis. Of course, there are other elements that are crucial to this process, for example, liberating the patient's mind so that free association can be relatively free. Some French analysts have put free association at the center of technique. Donnet (2001) noted that "in accordance with the project of an analytic cure, the method consists in carefully creating the conditions in which free association proves to be practical, interpretable, and beneficial" (p. 129). Green (2000) offered a similar view, "By constructing an analytic space in which free association and psychoanalytic listening are possible, the analyst can voice and link previously catastrophic ideas, quite unknown to the patient's consciousness, to help the patient to create meaning and obtain relief from previously dominant but unknown terrors" (p. 429).

There is a further issue to be considered. I believe a central principle of the analytic method is the necessity for the analyst to *identify and clarify* the psychical phenomenon before interpreting it. Consider the following simile. Think of a patient coming to us for help who speaks Russian, but who doesn't know he speaks Russian, and who doesn't understand Russian. We, on the other hand, have been trained to speak and understand "Russian". How would we begin to help this person? I think there would be general agreement that our first task would be to help them see they are speaking in a foreign language. This is our position as analysts. We first have to help the person see how their conscious language is conveying the language of the preconscious and unconscious. Qualities of the mind, universal in all patients (e.g., concrete thinking in the face of conflict), make this possible only in the *here and now*. To elaborate! In the midst of conflict, a patient's thinking is concrete. He can only see and think about what is immediately before his eyes (or ears). For long periods of time the patient is incapable of keeping a sequence of thoughts in mind while talking. Clinically we see evidence of this in that it is often only in the middle of treatment that we can make a surprise interpretation, capturing in a short form the essence of a reverie, and have some hope the patient will understand it in a non-intellectual fashion. What is missing earlier in treatment is the patient's capacity to follow his own thoughts and integrate them at a higher level of abstraction. Most analysts would agree that this is the level on which analysands are thinking through much of their analysis—they think, but do not think about their thinking. Piaget (1930) and Piaget and Inholder (1959) described this type of thinking as pre-operational. Others have described this type of thinking as "pre-symbolic" (Basch, 1981), "pre-conceptual" (Frosch, 1995), "concrete" (Bass, 1997; Busch, 1995, 2009; Frosch, 2011). What these labels attempt to capture is that the patient's thinking, at these times, is without *sufficient symbolic representations*. Inserting the word 'patient" for "child" we can see how accurately pre-operational thinking fits the thought processes of our patients through-out much of an analysis. Flavell (1963) states, *the child (patient)* "feels neither the compunction to justify his reasoning to others nor to look for possible contradictions in his logic. He is, for example, unable to reconstruct a chain of reasoning which he has just passed through; he thinks but he cannot think about his thinking" (p. 156). Flavell further describes thoughts that are considered "solely in terms of the phenom-enal, before-the-eye reality" (Flavell, 1963, p. 203). This is why through much of an analysis we need to work in the *here and now*. The *here and now is* the "before the eye reality". It is concrete; it is what *is* happening, it is not a speculation about something else. By working with what the patient is capable of thinking, we help him see how to think about thinking. *Premature use of metaphor or symbols in interpreting can lead to an iatrogenically induced intellectualization, confusion, and submission.*

Another Example

Sam: Back surgery necessitated that I had to interrupt working with patients for a month. I informed Sam of this approximately a month before, when I was first told of the necessity for surgery. Sam, age 45, was a successful businessman who hadn't been able to find a partner in spite of having no difficulty attracting women with whom he'd have short affairs. When he was six his parents divorced, after which he moved back and forth between his parents, each of whom had moved from the city where Sam lived, since he was born. As one can imagine my absence was particularly upsetting for Sam, although it wasn't a feeling he could be conscious of at the time. Shortly after my announcement of my time away, Sam started to miss appointments for "realistic" reasons. This eventually calmed down. The vignette I'll report took place a week before my surgery.

Sam: Well, I guess we won't be meeting much longer before your break. I'm thinking of going to a tennis camp for the first two weeks, but it really bugs me that I have to commit to be there the whole time. I plan to stay but you know how much I rebel against being forced to do anything. (Brief pause).

I had a dream where a child was hurt and crying, after he fell in a playground, and his mother was just gabbing away with other mothers. It was like my mother who seemed to spend her evenings talking on the phone, while me and my brother were left to watch whatever we wanted on television. She wasn't any better in the daytime. As soon as we'd come home from school, she would tell us to play outside, and was annoyed if we came in before dinner. This was after the divorce when I was six and my brother was four. It's interesting, I just remembered when I woke up from the dream, I thought of our appointment today.

FB: The first thing you mentioned when you started the session today was your awareness that we don't have much time before my back surgery, and my month absence from our work together. Given your association upon waking from the dream, it seems likely that while you consciously have little feeling about my absence, outside of awareness you seem to see me as being like your neglectful mother for my upcoming absence.

(In this interpretation, I'm using what comes to the patient's mind as the basis for interpreting his defense against experiencing me as neglectful for my absence. I'm emphasizing 'If we listen to what comes to your mind...' as a method that aids self-analysis.)

Sam: I can see that now.

FB: Maybe we can explore what *held back your awareness* that a part of you felt it is neglectful of me to, in essence, "force you" to take this month break.

Here I am focusing on the defense against his feelings that I'm being neglectful, while also pointing out the connection he's made in the dream with his neglectful mother. My focusing on the defense while also pointing to what is being defended against (i.e., a feeling that my absence matters) is possible because of his bringing up my upcoming absence, and his ability to remember the dream and bring it into the session indicating it is allowed into preconscious awareness rather than remaining unconscious.

Sam: It would mean I care about whether we meet or not. I don't know why that matters to me. Pause! I find myself thinking about this couple my wife invited for dinner this weekend. I'm excited because *he*, I mean *she* is very attractive. (Sam continue talking about all the ways he was very attracted to this woman.)

FB: I wonder if you noticed your slip when you began talking about your attraction to this woman, where instead of *she* you said *he*.

Sam: No, I didn't, but now that you reminded me of it, I did register it, but only barely.

FB: The slip came up after you were puzzled by why it matters to you whether you show you care if we meet or not. It seems to me that caring about whether we meet or not raises the specter of your attraction to a man, and the anxiety it arouses.

We had talked about this issue previously. His relationships with men were highly ambivalent. He would become close friends with a man, and after a while he'd flee the relationship based upon what he felt was a slight. Historically he seemed to have longed for his distant father to protect him from his over-stimulating, possessive mother.

From an early age, he sexualized most relationships.

Sam: That again. I see what you're saying but I find it very difficult to accept.

FB: I can see that, but I think it helps us understand why it's compli-cated for you to feel like your closeness to a man matters or not.

Sam: So, do you think this is one part of my convoluted relationships with men. Or is it me who's recognizing this and not wanting to own it at the same time.

In this example I think one can see how I'm following the Sam's associations, while bringing meaning to what these asso-ciations tell us about what's going on in his mind. I find when colleagues begin to learn my method, there is a tendency to just repeat the sequence of the patient's association, without giving the patient some clue as to why it's being brought to their atten-tion. While the implication in the analyst's mind is to see what comes to the patient's mind, but such clarifications often leave patients bewildered. It is clear the analyst is bringing this to the patient's attention for a reason, but it isn't clear why.

Specific Methods for Creating a Psychoanalytic Mind

There are certain changes in our methods of working that flow directly from the attempt to help the patient create a psychoanalytic mind and are central to the curative process. All have to do with how we enable the patient to build and accept new representations and bring what has been warded off and under-represented to preconscious aware-ness. Increasingly we have paid attention to the *manner in which we bring our observations and interpretations* to the patient's awareness, and the profound effect this has on the patient's ability to use what we say. It is another way of looking at the two-person nature of psy-choanalysis, while holding on to our understanding that it is the inner life of the patient we can help change. In what I'll describe, you will find the innovative ideas of psychoanalysts from different perspectives that have contributed to the *vitality* of contemporary psychoanalysis.[2]

Preconscious Thinking

We have moved from primarily confronting the patient with what the analyst gleans from the patient's unconscious, to working more closely with what the patient is able to hear, understand, and potentially integrate. In this way, we've realized that in order to help a patient grasp how they are ruled by unconscious fantasies, self-states, conflicts, etc., these have to first become understandable.[6]

Except for the French school, preconscious thinking has remained a 'shadow concept' (Busch, 2006), if a point of consideration at all. In fact, Green (1974) was one of the earliest proponents of the importance of the preconscious in our interpretive work. As I've noted previously (Busch, 2013), similar statements can be found in the diverse work of Paul Gray, Betty Joseph, Nino Ferro, and the Barangers. In 1915 Freud tried to *strictly* distinguish between unconscious and preconscious thinking on the basis of 'word presentations' and 'thing presentations'. However, buried in this paper is Freud's puzzlement over the fact that "A very great part of this preconscious originates in the unconscious, has the characteristics of its derivatives, and is subject to censorship before it can become conscious" (1915, p. 191), and that there are thoughts that had all the earmarks of having been formed *unconsciously*, "*but were highly organized, free from self-contradiction, have made use of every acquisition of the system Cs., and would hardly be distinguished in our judgment from the formations of that system*" (1915, p. 190, my italics).

Thus, in contrast to everything else he'd written in this paper, *Freud briefly conceives of complex preconscious thinking with infusions of unconscious elements.* In these few sentences, Freud, still in his Topographical Model, presents a view of *preconscious thinking that goes from a permeable border of the system Ucs to the permeable border of the system Cs.*[7]

If understood in this way, there are various levels of preconscious thinking at which we are working that make our task more complex. For example, the sexual derivatives that appear early in the treatment of a hysterical patient would be worked with differently compared to similar derivatives that appear in the later phases of an obsessional patient. While the hysterical patient's sexually tinged associations may seem like they are close to consciousness, they are more often closer to the unconscious border and hence more difficult to bring to awareness. The sexual derivatives in the obsessional's associations are more likely the result of the hard work of analyzing defenses, and thus more easily interpretable. As we are dealing with two different levels of psychic organization, *we adjust our interventions to the ego's* functioning, or to put it in Bionian terms, we metabolize for the patient what he can then further metabolize.

Building Representations

What is represented can continue to build structure and enhance the ability to contain psychic energies. This leads to what Green (1975) called "binding the inchoate" (p. 9) and containing it, thus giving a container to the patient's content and "content to his container" (p. 7).

Any time we name a vague something that was, as yet, unnamed we attempt to represent it with a word. Any time we discover and enhance *meaning* that previously resided in a suspended space, or capture meaning in a meaningful way to the patient, we are on the way to building a representation. The representation we build can be as delineated as a word, as complex as a metaphor, or as fleeting as an Ogden waking dream. Whether it becomes something that is representable for the analysand depends on many factors, *including how close it comes to what is tolerable at that exact clinical moment* (i.e., the patient's capacity to transform the elements of his familiar thinking into a new gestalt). After each intervention we see what the patient can make of it at that moment. We can call it the work of the alpha function or his ego function. *Decisive is whether the patient can allow our interventions to work on his mind.* Representations are not absent or present but are there in a variety of forms. In broad brushstrokes, when we talk about building representations in psychoanalysis, we are talking about separate but related issues. The first is building a more nuanced, complex representation out of a highly saturated, simple one. The second is developing a beginning representation from its more primitive, non-symbolic representational origins. Further, one can think of representations as having multiple dimensions: They may range from deeply unconscious to close to the **preconscious** from simple to complex with varying degrees of saturation. In this model, building representations means attempting to make representations more complex, bring them closer to consciousness, and make them less saturated (or more nuanced). For example, at times we try to build a representation from one that is conceptually primitive (e.g., somatic representations). With a rigid, highly saturated, simple representation that is close to consciousness (i.e., all men are animals, ego psychology is superficial), we attempt to make the representation more complex and less saturated (e.g., some men **can be authoritarian and try to dominate**).

Free associations: What I most often say to a patient is based on their associations. I agree with the French analyst Marilia Aisenstein (2009), who stated, "In my view, the opening up and enrichment of thought processes in analysis, with the help of the method of free association (which permits integration of unconscious movements into secondary processes) is the greatest therapeutic effect of the psychoanalytic cure" (p. 896). In fact, as early as 1939, Hartman noted the significance of *linking representations*, more so than reconstruction, in moving the analysis forward. He felt that the interpretive emphasis on reconstruction, while important, should not take precedence over *"instances in which the causal connections of elements, and the criteria for these connections, are established"* (Hartmann, 1939, p. 63, italics added).

Further, it's my view that in one form or another, everything that happens in an analytic session is a free association, and all we need to know can be found in the patient's free associations. In the patient's use of the method of free association, we can see how unknown thoughts guide her, inhibit her, and destroy her. We can also come to understand the process by which patients guide, inhibit, and destroy their thoughts. Sometimes thoughts are told in words, sometimes in the absence of words. As mentioned earlier sometimes they are more like actions. There are some analysts who believe all speech is action, but I think most analysts would agree that we can differentiate between when a patient's speech is a linked set of associations, and when language is taken over by action leading to the analyst's countertransference feelings.

Interpreting 'In the Neighborhood' (Busch, 1993)

Freud first articulated this principle when he warned a young physician about the uselessness of *wild interpretations*, by which he meant interpretations the patient wasn't ready for:

If knowledge about the unconscious were as important for the patient as people inexperienced in psycho-analysis imagine, listening to lectures or reading books would be enough to cure him. Such measures, however, have as much influence on the symptoms of nervous illness as a distribution of menu-cards in a time of famine has upon hunger ... Since, however, psycho-analysis cannot dispense with giving this information, it lays down that this shall not be done before the patient must, through preparation, himself have *reached the neighborhood of what he has repressed.*

(1910, pp. 225–226, italics added)

By introducing the concept of the analysand needing to be "in the neighborhood", Freud is noting, amongst all the principles of clinical technique, the *centrality of the preconscious*. No matter how brilliant the analyst's reading of the unconscious, it is not useful data until it can be connected to something the patient can be preconsciously aware of.[11]

Listening to discussions of the clinical process, one is impressed with how many interpretations seem based *less on what the patient is capable of hearing*, and more on what the analyst is capable of understanding. Maybe it's only that the presenter didn't bring the audience into the neighborhood of what he did, but maybe we too often confuse our ability to read the unconscious with the patient's ability to understand it. We are frequently not clear enough on the distinction between an unconscious communication and our ability to communicate with the patient's unconscious. What the patient can hear, understand, and effectively utilize—let alone the benefits of considering such an approach—are only gradually entering the foreground of our clinical discussions.

Green explained it this way:

> I support the Freudian concept of the ego in which the patient's freedom is respected and *which allows one to proceed according to what the patient is able to understand of what we are saying to him at that point in time of the treatment*, i.e., permitting him to elaborate and integrate in a regression-progression process, and so to proceed from the most superficial to the deepest level.
>
> (1974, p. 421)

In fact, as I've noted previously (Busch, 2013), analysts from widely varying theoretical perspectives (e.g., Ferro, 2003, pp. 189–190; Baranger, 1993, p. 23; Ikonen, 2003, p. 5; Bion, 1962, p. 87) are increasingly attentive to the ways we think about the "neighborhood" as a guide to the patient's capacity to understand and utilize an intervention in an emotionally and cognitively meaningful manner, and the ways the analyst functions that may foster or hinder this process.

Clarification

Edward Bibring's (1954) introduction of this concept never received traction as a defined method of psychoanalytic technique. I think it was because in his writing, he limited the use of clarification to material that was close to consciousness. However, in reading the examples he provides, what he describes are actually *clarifications of derivatives of unconsciously motivated thinking that are preconsciously organized*. This latter way is an important use of clarification, as well as the need to clarify the patient's unconscious use of words as actions. This differs from an *interpretation*, where we try to raise *unconscious meaning* to awareness. Betty Joseph emphasizes a similar process when she suggests the elucidation of those ways in which the patient,for example, creates tone and atmosphere for understanding or against understanding. She argues that only when this is *clarified*, which often takes repeated demonstrations, is it helpful to move toward understanding the reasons or motives for such behavior.

The reason for the need for clarification is simple—in the midst of conflict, a patient's thinking is concrete (Busch, 1995, 2009).[12] He can only think[13] about what is immediately present. For long periods of time, and even when the patient is freely associating, he is incapable of keeping track of the sequence of his thoughts while talking. It requires a great deal of time before we can make an interpretation that may be a word, or metaphor, capturing in a short form the essence of a reverie, and have some hope the patient will understand it in a non-intellectual fashion. What is missing earlier in treatment is the patient's capacity to follow his own thoughts and integrate them at a higher level of abstraction (Busch, 1995, 2009).[14] Most analysts would agree that this is the level on which an analysand is functioning through much of his analysis—*he thinks, but he cannot think about his thinking*. Thus, in order to make progress, the patient needs to experience an interpretation, but to do this we need to *clarify* what he's been doing or saying that led to our interpretation.

Countertransference

The discovery of the importance of *countertransference* thoughts and feelings as a crucial source of information in the psychoanalytic situation has been one of our most significant advances. Beginning with the pioneering work of the Kleinians on projective identification and followed by so many others, we've come to realize its significance in understanding every patient *at some point* in their analysis, and its importance in understanding other patients from the moment they walk into our consulting room. After a time of fierce debate, change took place, and now I know of no theory that dismisses the importance of countertransference feelings in understanding our patients.

However, we also need to heed Hanna Segal's (Hunter, 1993) warning that countertransference *is our best servant and worst master*. As essential as it is as a tool in our analytic work, *it also provides data that is difficult to sort out and translate*. In response to the patient, we may grow anxious, impatient, or withdrawn. If we have a psychoanalytic mind, we can notice and reflect on these occurrences, without having to act, while recognizing that a certain amount of acting on our countertransference is inevitable (and sometimes useful in understanding).

A particular problem that analysts face is that we often feel forced by the patient into what seems like an alien position, which can drive us to push back and *force the patient to accept his own unconscious.* At these times, the countertransference interpretation seems to result from a wish to expel what is transferred back onto the patient. "You feel this way, not me", we seem to be saying, while meaning to be exploratory or interpretive. It is a way of the analyst getting rid of something uncomfortable stirred in his own unconscious.[15] Another problem we face is when we seem to treat our countertransference reactions as an *unerring guides to the patient's behavior*—what I call "the Descartian Somersault" (i.e., I think, therefore you are). Further, it can be a formulaic way of warding off deeper, more conflicted feelings, which is understandable given that countertransference reactions are first registered unconsciously.

In the face of a countertransference reaction, it takes considerable restraint, narcissistic balance, and an ongoing self-analytic capacity to maintain our role of empathic and reflective participant-observer and forestall the pull towards enactment. Without a capacity for introspection and self-inquiry about these countertransference feelings, it is difficult to see how one could sort out these unique moments created by the two participants.

Interpsychic Communication

Bolognini (2011) introduced the term *interpsychic* to capture the conscious and unconscious dialogue of two interacting people—patient and analyst—"a territory for which we have only barely been able to find words—despite all the words that are in use for it" (Schmidt-Hellerau, 2011, p. 447). Diamond (2014) shows the contributions and acceptance of this term, *interpsychic*, from a wide variety of psychoanalytic cultures (although not labeled as such). In short, this term *interpsychic* broadens the field for the analyst to include a number of states of mind, often thought of as separate, to both understand the patient and demonstrate, without teaching, how the analyst is thinking. In working with the interior of one's mind in response to the patient, there are important ethical and clinical considerations that aren't always noted.

Diamond warns,

As with every technical innovation, especially the current emphasized use of the analyst's mental experience, there is an ever-present danger of misuse as well as possible ethical transgressions. When taken to extreme, this can lead away from the patient's psychology and center on the analyst's or the dyadic process per se.

(2014, p. 531)

Therefore, it is wise to keep in mind that this method is only part of our analytic technique. We need to listen to the analysand and ourselves polyphonically to appreciate *how best to listen*. Finally, how we translate our inner thoughts into usable interpretations is something that is still to be fully understood.

Analyst-Centered Interpretations

Steiner (1994) introduced an important clinical term—"analyst-centered interpretations"—for working with more disturbed patients where "The priority for the patient is to get rid of unwanted mental contents, which he projects into the analyst. In these states he is able to take very little back into his mind" (1994, p. 406). He goes on to say that the patient feels threatened if the analyst continues to tell him what he (the patient) is thinking or feeling, as this is what is projected into the analyst as a way of getting rid of these feelings. I would suggest this is in sync with a solid ego psychological position where the paranoid-schizoid patient's regressed ego functions are taken into consideration.

I would add that *analyst-centered interpretations* are useful in the full spectrum of pathologies, especially early in the treatment, and throughout the treatment when new regressions emerge. This is because all of our patients are dealing with unconscious thoughts and feelings that are terrifying to know about, as they are associated in the patient's unconscious mind with the most frightening terrors known to man. Therefore, any way we can work to ease these terrors while analyzing them will benefit the patient.

Learning from Steiner's basic idea but modifying it from his work with borderline and psychotic patients within a Kleinian perspective, I have often found the following approach central to help patients open their minds to a new way of thinking of themselves. The basic premise of the method is to *wonder with the patient about the analyst's impressions rather than telling the patient they are something, or what she's truly feeling or thinking*. This latter way seems more common in clinical practice, as when the analyst says, "You are angry at me, and cannot tolerate it, so you imagine me as angry". An analyst-centered approach seems to help the patient observe something about herself without the sense of being told she *is* a particular way, which may be harder to internalize in the early phase of treatment as it can often bring a severe super-ego reaction. This is especially true with moments that are clearly important but are more difficult for the patient to observe because of their ineffable quality. Later in treatment, an analyst-centered interpretation is useful when something unconscious is about to emerge, which, if addressed too directly, would lead to it being repressed again.

Language Action

First identified by Freud (1914), this concept captures a patient's way of talking that is unconsciously meant to *do something*. At these times, words become attempts to bore, seduce, anger, or excite the analyst. This was evocatively captured by McLaughlin when he stated that words "become acts, things—sticks and stones, hugs and holdings" (1991, p. 598). While it seems like the patient is describing a dream, recalling an upsetting event, or complaining about a spouse, the analyst feels mocked for his interest in dreams, blamed for the patient's bad luck, or faced with a demand for unconditional love.[17]

We've been aware of the *consequences* of language action for some time, as it often leads to the analyst's countertransference reaction. However, the *significance of clarifying how language action is expressed before identifying its effects or its unconscious meaning* has only become evident more recently (Busch, 2009, 2013; Joseph, 1985). We can hear this approach in Feldman's (2004) description of Joseph's work when he says that her assumption is "that real psychic change is more likely to be promoted by the detailed description of how the patient is using the analyst, using interpretations, or using her mind in a given session, and then to move on to the way the patient's history, and unconscious phantasies express themselves in the immediacy of the processes and interactions in the session" (Feldman, 2004, p. 28).

That is, we try to understand what a patient is *doing with* us in their words, tone, phrasing of sentences, and ideas expressed. Once we recognize our countertransference reaction to language action and reflect upon it, this action has already begun to be transformed, that is, represented within the mind of the analyst. From here the analyst can translate the language action into words, which gives the patient increasing degrees of freedom to think and feel.

It is important to remember that the entire range of psychic states can be expressed in language action. My sense is that in our countertransference reaction to language action, we've overemphasized what the patient is doing to the analyst, rather than what he might also be doing for himself (e.g., repairing a fragile self-state).

I end this chapter with what I believe is one of the most important statements about the method of psychoanalysis (Green, 1974), which I've elaborated on in my own way, as I've discussed above.

The analysis of the preconscious and in particular the use of the patient's analytical material (in his own language) has been neglected since Freud. The reason for this appears to be straightforward in that, since the preconscious can be reached by the conscious, the importance of the preconscious is negligible and language is superficial. To me, however, this viewpoint is superficial itself. The preconscious, as we have seen, is a privileged space where both the analyst and the patient can meet to share part of the transference and go forward together. There is no point in the analyst running like a hare if the patient moves like a tortoise. A meeting point in depth is more probable if the thread that links the two travelers also serves to keep them sufficiently apart.

(p. 421)

In the analytic situation there are two alternatives: "either the analyst uses the preconscious as a mediator and continues the analytical work towards the unconscious by following the route of communications from the preconscious to the conscious, aware of trying to reach the unconscious by this well-worn path, in which case resistances will slowly give way, inflicting the ego with only minor traumas; or else he goes directly from the conscious to the unconscious causing a real narcissistic wound, due to the method employed for interpreting, rather than to the content of the interpretation. In this case, needless to say, the patient can react to this intrusion only in an unfavourable way—either by a protective denial of his inner space, or by complacently accepting a false self and without really believing in it or, again, by building up a masochistic type of therapeutic alliance: "Give me more interpretations, rape me, hurt me, I like it". This leads to an erotization of the superego, cheating it of its own nature. The rule that one should interpret as near as possible to the ego is justified if one does not wish to foster the establishment of a cement block of resistances which characterizes the beginning of interminable analyses. It is indeed noticeable that analyses which right from the start involve lengthy and frequent interpretations are hardly ever shorter than the others; indeed, it is quite the contrary.

(pp. 416–417)

Notes

1 See Busch (2000) for an elaboration on this point.
2 I have identified these methods previously in Busch, 2013, 2015.

References

Aisenstein, M. (2009) Discussion of Sander M. Abend's "Freud, Transference, and Therapeutic Action". *Psychoanalytic Quarterly*. 78:893-901
Baranger, M. (1993) The Mind of the Analyst: From Listening to Interpretation. *International Journal of Psychoanalysis*. 74:15–24.

Bibring, E. (1954) Psychoanalysis and the Dynamic Psychotherapies. *Journal of the American Psychoanalytic Association.* 2:745–770.

Bion, W.R. (1962) *Learning from Experience.* London: Tavistock.

Bolognini, S. (2011) *Secret Passages.* London: Routledge.

Busch, F. (1993) In the Neighborhood: Aspects of a Good Interpretation and a "Developmental Lag" in Ego Psychology. *Journal of the American Psychoanalytic Association.* 41:151–76.

Busch, F. (1995) Do Actions Speak Louder than Words? A Query into an Enigma in Psychoanalytic Theory and Technique. *Journal of the American Psychoanalytic Association.* 43:61–82.

Busch, F. (2000) What is a Deep Interpretation?. *Journal of the American Psychoanalytic Association.* 48: 237-254

Busch, F. (2006) A Shadow Concept. *International Journal of Psychoanalysis.* 87:1471–1485.

Busch, F. (2009) Can you Push a Camel Through the Eye of a Needle? *International Journal of Psychoanalysis.* 90:53–68.

Busch, F. (2013) -*Creating a Psychoanalytic Mind.* London: Routledge.

Diamond, M. (2014) Analytic Mind use and Interpsychic Communication. *Psychoanalytic Quarterly* 83:525–564.

Donnet, J. (2001) From the Fundamental Rule to the Analysing Situation. *International Journal of Psychoanalysis* 82:129–140.

Feldman, M. (2004) Supporting Psychic Change: Betty Joseph. In Hargreaves, E. and Varchekver, A. (eds.), *In Pursuit of Psychic Change*, 20–35. London: Routledge.

Feldman, M. (2007) The Illumination of History. *International Journal of Psychoanalysis* 88:609–625.

Ferro, N. (2003) Marcella: The Transition from Explosive Sensoriality to the Ability to Think. *Psychoanalytic Quarterly* 72:183–200.

Flavell, J.H. (1963) *The Developmental Psychology of Jean Piaget.* Princreton, NJ: Van Nostrand.

Freud, S. (1910) "Wild" Psycho-analysis. *S.E.* XI: 221–227.

Freud, S. (1914) Remembering, Repeating, and Working Through. *S.E.* XII:145–156.

Freud, S. (1915) The Unconscious. *S.E.* XIV:159–215.

Freud, S. (1931) Letter from Sigmund Freud to Stefan Zweig, February 7, 1931. Letters of Sigmund Freud 1873–1939 51:402–403.

Frosch, A. (1995) The Preconceptual Organizations of Emotions. *Journal of the American Psychoanalytic Association.* 43: 423-447.

Green, A. (1974) Surface Analysis, Deep Analysis (The Role of the Preconscious in Psychoanalytical Technique). *International Review of Psychoanalysis* 1:415–423.

Green, A. (1975) The Analyst, Symbolization, and Absence in the Analytic Setting (On Changes in Analytic Practice and Analytic Experience): In Memory of D. W. Winnicott. *International Review of Psychoanalysis* 56:1–22.

Green, A. (2000) The Central Phobic Position: A New Formulation of the Free Association Method. *International Journal of Psychoanalysis* 81:429–451.

Hartmann, H. (1939) *The Ego and the Problem of Adaptation.* New York International University Press. (English version 1958)

Hunter, V. (1993) An Interview with Hanna Segal. *Psychoanalytic Review* 80(1):1–28.

Ikonen, P. (2003) A Few Reflections on How We May Approach the Unconscious. *Scandinavian Psychoanalytic Review* 26:3–10.

Kris, A. (1982). *Free Association.* New York: International University Press.

Joseph, B. (1985) Transference: The Total Situation. *International Journal of Psychoanalysis* 66:447–454.

McLaughlin, J.T. (1991) Clinical and Theoretical Aspects of Enactment. *Journal of the American Psychoanalytic Association* 39:595–614.

Ogden, T. (2007). On Talking as Dreaming.*International Journal of Psychoanalysis.* 88: 575-589.

Schacter, J. (1992), Concepts of termination and post-termination patient-analyst contact. *International Journal of Psychoanalysis.* 73: 137-154.

Schacter, J. (1992), Concepts of termination and post-termination patient-analyst contact. *International Journal of Psychoanalysis.* 73: 137-154.

Schmidt-Hellerau, C. (2011) Secret Passages: Review of Bolognini's book. *Psychoanalytic Quarterly* 81:443–455.

Steiner, J. (1994) Patient-centered and Analyst-centered Interpretations: Some Implications of Containment and Countertransference. *Psychoanalytic Inquiry* 14:406–422.

3 Discovering Self-Analysis

Within a Freudian Framework

The capacity for self-analysis has been a staple of psychoanalytic treatment since Freud's self-analysis led to the discovery of his own unconscious. In a letter to Flies (1897), Freud wrote, "My self-analysis is in fact the most essential thing I have at present, and it promises to become of the greatest value to me if it reaches its end". Many years later, Fine (1979) took the position that "It was the self-analysis which allowed Freud to take the decisive steps forward in his psychology. Hence it is the self-analysis which should be looked upon as the real seed from which psychoanalysis grew" (p. 20). In fact, at the beginning of the 20th century, Abraham, Ferenczi, Jones, and Jung all wrote to Freud about their self-analysis. Yet, throughout the vast literature on self-analysis, *there are very few descriptions of what processes are necessary in analysis for self-analysis to develop.* In this chapter, after a brief survey of the literature, I will present ways of analyzing that, I believe, lead the analysand to *discover the process of analysis leading to the capacity for self-analysis. Self-analysis, as an analytic goal, is a crucial aspect of any analysis, as no analysis is ever complete. In order to deal with variations that can develop on what had previously been discovered in one's analysis, or when new conflicts develop as life continues, the capacity for self-analysis can lead to new discoveries instead of relying on previous interpretations from a prior analysis. Self-analysis can also become an exhilarating part of everyday life, as one can find interesting and funny connections in the ongoing soliloquy in one's mind.* If this phase can be reached, it signifies the beginning of the termination phase, and the resistances against it, which are a significant part of the path to self-analysis (e.g., see Busch, (2013, pp. 148–158).

By the 1930s, doubts had begun to develop about the capacity for self-analysis. Near the end of his life, in a short note on a parapraxis (1935), Freud remarked in passing: "In self-analysis the danger of incompleteness is particularly great. One is too soon satisfied with a part explanation, behind which resistance may easily be keeping back something that is more important perhaps" (p. -234). This warning was repeated by Freud in 1939. Both Bibring (1952) and Obendorf

DOI: 10.4324/9781032658704-5

(1954) put forth the idea that the problem with self-analysis was the countertransference.

From the 1900s on, there were hundreds and sometimes thousands of references to self-analysis every decade (the total from PEP-web was over 5,000), but *rarely was there a discussion of how self-analysis came about*. It seemed as if it was supposed to be the end-product of a "good enough" analysis. Ultimately, this idea was put forward by Windholz (1955), who, in describing analyses of candidates, believed that "The aim of the didactic analysis is to prepare the candidate for self-analysis" (p. 658), a point echoed in a slightly different form by Meltzer (1967). Windholz goes on to say that "The therapeutic effectiveness of the analysis should protect the analyst from interferences originating in his own unconscious" (pp. 658–659). Windholz was also one of the first to put forth the idea that *identification with the analyst's way of analyzing is an important part of self-analysis*. "The *candidate* identifies with this attitude which furthers the development of the ego's capacity to tolerate derivatives of unconscious impulses under the benevolent yet continuous scrutiny of an analytic super-ego" (p. 649). Kramer (1959) continued this line of thinking when he wrote, "The positive transference as an incentive to face inner conflicts is replaced by superego and ego-ideal demand and approval. This replacement takes place through identification with the analyst" (p. 18). This echoed a much earlier paper by Strachey (1934) on the mutative interpretation, where he put forth the idea that it was the analyst's benevolent superego that allowed patients to accept interpretations.

The concept of self-analysis continued to be explored, with *variations on the belief of the importance of the analysand's identification with the analyst*. Rangell, in a panel (Firestein, 1969), proclaimed that by incorporating into the ego the *analytic functions* of the analyst, self-analysis can survive the transference neurosis and continue into the post-analytic phase. In a later elaboration, Rangell (1979) suggested that it's a constant series of micro-identifications (Kohut's "transmuting internalizations") with the analyzing function of the analyst that enables analysis to take place, first partially and experimentally, then with more familiarity and sureness, and, finally, with an autonomy which one hopes will continue with self-analysis afterward. Grinberg (1980, p. 27) also captured an element of the thinking during this time when he stated:

I believe that analysis does not terminate with the separation of the analyst and the analysand. The only thing which ends is the relationship between them, giving way to a new phase of continuation of the process through self-analysis ... In other words, the psychoanalytic relationship is terminated, or is about to end, when the *psychoanalytic process has been internalized by the analysand*.

(p. 27, italics added)

Schafer (1979), describing psychoanalytic methods for changes in character, wrote:

> this kind of change that is meant when one speaks of genuine insight and of the development through analysis of a continuing capacity for self-analysis. Thus, late in effective analyses and in post-analytic sessions, one sees analysands still beginning to create or accept crises of the old sort and then catching themselves in the act, questioning what they are up to—that is, asking themselves how they are threatened and why—and then going on to consider alternative views of their situations and the courses of action open to them—all of which, taken together, would have been unthinkable during early stages of their analyses.
>
> (p. 886)

The few studies of analytic outcome support Schafer's position. Follow-up studies of completed psychoanalyses (Schlessinger and Robbins, 1983) make it evident that conflicts are not obliterated, resolved, or any of the other previously used terms which suggested that analysis did away with conflict.

> What has become clearer is that even after analysis, conflicts remain alive and ready elements in an individual's psyche. What changes is an individual's ability to respond to the arousal of conflicts in a more adaptive manner. Some process of ongoing self-analysis occurs, which allows the individual's ego to respond in new situations of conflict arousal in a more flexible fashion.
>
> (ibid., p. 866)

The most striking result to come out of the Stockholm outcome studies, probably the most comprehensive research on psychoanalysis and psychotherapy (Falkenström et al., 2007), was the significance of self-analysis in treatment gains. That is, *psychoanalytic patients develop the capacity for self-analysis while psychotherapy patients tend not to, and this was responsible for the significantly different post-termination gains in the psychoanalytic group.* This confirmed the earlier findings of Leuzinger-Bohleber et al. (2003) and Kantrowitz et al. (1990). These powerful research findings confirm what has always been an argument for the benefits of psychoanalysis, that is, the analysand's ongoing capacity to profit from self-analysis to deal with the exigencies of life. A more skeptical view was presented by Kramer (1959) at an earlier time:

> I feel certain that every analyst who has tried to continue analyzing himself has had the experience of encountering insurmountable

resistances. At such times, dreams are forgotten, and associations remain fruitless. Interpretations are tentative, they prove to be wrong or sterile intellectual speculations. Any insight that might occur is apt to be about a minor matter and does not lead to a resolution of the conflict. Superego promptings to continue the analytic efforts lead to further awareness of the frustrating power of the resistances. One often has to admit defeat.

(p. 19)[1]

Kernberg (2007) cogently argued that a "core issue for narcissistic patients is their inability to depend on the therapist, because such dependency is experienced as humiliating. Such fear of dependency, often unconscious, is defended against with attempts to omnipotently control the treatment" (Rosenfeld, 1987). Clinically, this takes the form of the patient's efforts at "self-analysis," as opposed to a collaboration with the therapist leading to integration and reflection.

These patients treat the therapist as if he were a 'vending machine' of interpretations, which they then appropriate as their own, at the same time being chronically disappointed for not receiving enough interpretations, or not the right kind, unconsciously dismissing everything they might learn from him. For this reason, treatment often maintains a 'first session' quality over an extended period. Narcissistic patients show themselves as intensely competitive with the therapist and are suspicious of what they consider his indifferent or exploitative attitude toward them. They cannot conceive the therapist as spontaneously interested and honestly concerned about them; as a result, they evince significant devaluation and contempt of the therapist.

(p. 506)

Discovering Self-Analysis

For many years, it has been my impression that an analysand needs to *discover* a way of analyzing that leads to self-analysis, and that *this depends on certain ways the analyst analyzes*. But first, what do I mean by self-analysis? In my view, it means using the *analytic method* as I understand it, that is seeing what comes to mind and then reflecting upon it with an open mind. It sounds deceptively simple, but it often takes a long time in analysis for the analysand to discover its importance. Once discovered, there is usually a period of excitement when the patient is finding his own mind. The analysand can, at times, find pleasure in his mind and play with ideas. This is often followed by resistances and regressions that need to be understood. This is one of the most important parts of the termination phase. It requires the analyst to follow ways of working described in Chapter 3 and elsewhere (e.g., Busch, 2013). In brief, it requires analyzing the patient's way of analyzing and repeated demonstrations of the analyst using the patient's thoughts as the basis of his interventions.[2]

Simon

Whatever instructions we give to patients in starting analysis, inevitably the analysand will develop a way of analyzing that fits some dynamic need. For example, Simon, a 45-year-old successful businessman, would bring in a dream every session, and then "associate" to it in a way that I characterized to myself as "paint by numbers". He had been in a previous analysis, where it seemed the transference was emphasized by the analyst and Simon's "associations" to dreams seemed to echo genetic formulations that Simon appeared to receive from his former analysts. In my own mind, I started to think that Simon clung to a way of working with his previous analyst so that he didn't engage with my way of doing analysis. In one session, Simon began in a typical fashion.

Simon: I had a dream last night. There was this guy who was walking in front of me, and I wanted to see this guy ... (pause) ... and talk to him and it looked like he didn't want to talk to me. (I noticed the pause, and it is often something I might ask about as it seemed like something was happening in his mind that interrupted his associations, but since this was the beginning of the session, I waited to see what would follow. I usually don't say anything at the beginning of a session so that I can see where the patient's mind takes him.)

Simon: (continuing) and so I think *obviously* this guy in the front was you and I was the other guy. I think this probably goes back to my mother and father who I felt were angry with me.

(FB's thoughts) There is a lot going on in this opening, with important transference implications. However, I thought the most important element was his *way of analyzing*, which was to quickly come to conclusions that seemed questionable. For example, saying "obviously" the guy in front was me (FB), when it wasn't obvious to me. I was thinking that he reversed our positions in the analysis, and I noted how he linked his parents anger with me. While I could have interpreted this content, I believed it was more important to clarify *his way of analyzing*. This was because even if he gained some greater understanding of the content, it would have been used by him in his characteristic style of "analyzing", which seemed to be an on-going enactment.

FB: As we've talked about before, it's my impression that in dealing with the dream you come up with answers rather than seeing what you may find.

Simon: I know we talked about this before, but this is what's coming to mind.

FB: I appreciate that, and now it seems important *why* that way of thinking about the dream came to mind rather than another.

There was a brief pause, and then Simon talked about how the previous evening he sent his sister an email suggesting that if she wanted to see a therapist, he would pay for it.

(I remembered that he offered this to his sister numerous times, along with money, and this usually angered her.)

FB: It was my impression that when you offered this in the past, it often made your sister angry (to which he agrees). Making someone angry comes up as a thought in response to why you may be interpreting dreams in the way you do.

Simon first talked about the rational reasons he offered his sister help; for example, the fact that she's not eating, her previous anorexia, and several others. He then said when previously he talked with me about all her problems and he thought about suggesting therapy and he decided against it, he then thought when I asked "Why?" (which I didn't remember asking), *he thought I was suggesting that he should have offered to pay for her therapy,* and that's why he brought it up.

His thoughts then went to when he was about 13 or 14, and he had this great counselor at summer camp (Barry).

Simon: He was really cool. He was also the basketball coach. There was this one game where we played against another, much bigger camp, and I was amazing. I scored 40 points and we beat them. I've always had the thought that it was Barry that caused me to score all these points. He did something like gave me a special incentive or told the other players to give me the ball, but he didn't remember anything like that actually happening. (I then remembered a story he told me earlier where he became a star baseball player in high school and believed his father had done something, like talked to the other coaches or umpires to make it happen.) He then brings in an incident with his wife. On the previous day he was thinking it would be nice to take a walk with her and imagined some things to talk about. She then came into his study and suggested they take a walk and he got pissed. He sounds angry when he says, "She's taking over" (a constant theme).

FB: *If we follow your thoughts* it seems like a part of you longs for someone to guide, support, and ease the way for you. Yet when your wife offers you exactly what you imagined, it makes you angry and you feel intruded upon.

Simon: When I was in analysis with Harold, I thought he was suggesting I do certain things, like getting married and having children. I did get married but never had children.

In this session, one can follow how I first point to Simon's *way of analyzing* and clarify it without suggesting any reason for why this is happening. He then associates emailing his sister with his paying for therapy, as he thought I had suggested. This seemed to be part of a central fantasy of having been secretly guided by a man so that he could stand out. I then clarify that and point to his ambivalence about it. At a later time, Simon's ambivalence around looking to a man to guide him led us to understand his fear/excitement in response to homosexual fantasies. As the analysis continued, we discovered an unconscious fantasy of being anally raped by a strong older man but stealing the man's penis to make him (Simon) bigger.

In this session, there are two ways of analyzing that are central to the possibility of the analysand engaging in self-analysis. The first is that the patient's way of analyzing needs to be clarified and then interpreted. Further, there has to be a connection between the patient's associations and the analyst's interventions. In this way, the patient eventually understands that it's what is coming to his mind that is the *data of analysis*, rather than searching for previous interpretations from his former analyst or from me to try and explain away troubling thoughts and feelings.

In summary, no analysis is ever complete, and there will be times in every analysand's life when a new conflict, or one not fully analyzed, will come to the fore. It is at these times when the capacity for self-analysis is crucial in determining the resolution or not of the burgeoning conflict. In my way of thinking, the development of the capacity for self-analysis is dependent on:

1. Clarifying and analyzing the patient's way of analyzing.
2. The patient's associations as the basic data of analysis.
3. Analyzing according to the principles described as *working in the neighborhood.*
4. *Working through the inevitable resistances to free association and roaming in one's mind during the termination.*

Notes

1   An oddity I found difficult to explain was that up until around 2000, by far the greatest majority of articles were written by analysts from America. Those analysts who had the greatest impact on European and Latin American analysts, Bion, Klein, and Winnicott, made no references to self-analysis in their work. However, it was the post-Bionians. that is Rochas de Barros, Ogden, Ferro, Levine, Brown, and many others. who

have written a great deal about the importance of self-analysis in their work. As I've written previously (Busch, 2019), I have many questions about what some of the post-Bionians consider self-analysis.

2 In supervision, I've seen how when introduced to my method of working, supervisees often start an intervention by reporting back to the patient exactly what he said. However, what I try to do is try to use the *essence* of what the patient said so it is recognizable to him, while including the emotional shading that accompanies it.

References

Bibring, G.L. (1952) 103rd Bulletin of the International Psycho-Analytical Association—Report on the Seventeenth International Psycho-Analytical Congress. *Bulletin of the International Psycho-Analytical Association* 33:249–272.

Busch, F. (1993) "In the Neighborhood": Aspects of a Good Interpretation and a "Developmental Lag" in Ego Psychology. *Journal of the American Psychoanalytic Association* 41:151–177.

Busch, F. (2013) *Creating a Psychoanalytic Mind*. London: Routledge.

Busch, F. (2019) *The Analyst's Reveries: An Exploration of Bion's Enigmatic Concept*. London: Routledge.

Falkenström, F., Grant, J., Broberg, B. and Sandell, R. (2007) Self-analysis and Post-termination Improvement After Psychoanalysis and Long-term Therapy. *Journal of the American Psychoanalytic Association* 55:529–673.

Fine, R. (1979) L'Auto-Analyse De Freud et la Découverte De La Psychanalyse Freud's Self-Analysis and the Discovery of Psychoanalysis. Didier Anzieu. Presses Universitaires de France, 1975, 853 pp. In 2 vols. with Photographic Supplement. *Psychoanalytic Review* 66:617–620.

Firestein, S.K. (1969) Problems of Termination in the Analysis of Adults. *Journal of the American Psychoanalytic Association* 17:222–237.

Freud, S. (1897) Letter 71 Extracts from the Fliess Papers. *S.E.* 1:263–266.

Freud, S. (1935) The Subtleties of a Faulty Action. *S.E.* 22:231–236.

Freud, S. (1939) The Fineness of Parapraxiz. *Psychoanalytic Review* 26:153–154.

Grinberg, L. (1980) The Closing Phase of the Psychoanalytic Treatment of Adults and the Goals of Psychoanalysis: "The Search for Truth About Oneself". *International Journal of Psychoanalysis* 61:25–37.

Kantrowitz, J., Katz, A.L. and Paolitto, F. (1990) Follow-up of Psychoanalysis Five to the Years After Termination: II. Development of the Self-analytic Function. *Journal of the American Psychoanalytic Association* 38:637–654.

Kernberg, O.F. (2007) The Almost Untreatable Narcissistic Patient. *Journal of the American Psychoanalytic Association* 55:503–539.

Kramer, M.K. (1959) On the Continuation of the Analytic Process After Psycho-Analysis (A Self-Observation). *International Journal of Psychoanalysis* 40:17–25.

Leuzinger-Bohleber, M., Stuhr, U., Rueger, B. and Beutel, M. (2003) How to Study the 'Quality of Psychoanalytic Treatments' and Their Long-term Effect on Patients' Well-being. *International Journal of Psychoanalysis* 84:263–290.

Leuzinger-Bohleber, M., Stuhr, U., Rueger, B. and Beutel, M. (2003) How to Study the 'Quality of Psychoanalytic Treatments' and Their Long-term Effect on Patients' Well-being. *International Journal of Psychoanalysis* 84:263–290.

Meltzer, D. (1967) *The Psychoanalytic Process*. London: William Heinemann Medical Books Ltd.

Rangell, L. (1979) Contemporary Issues in the Theory of Therapy. Contemporary Issues in the Theory of Therapy. *Journal of the American Psychoanalytic Association* 27:81–112.

Rosenfeld, H. (1987) *Impasse and Interpretation: Therapeutic and Anti-Therapeutic Factors in the Psychoanalytic Treatment of Psychotic, Borderline, and Neurotic Patients*. London: New Library of Psychoanalysis.

Schafer, R. (1979) Character, Ego-Syntonicity, and Character Change. *Journal of the American Psychoanalytic Association* 27:867–891.

Schlessinger, N. and Robbins, F.P. (1983) *A Developmental View of the Psychoanalytic Process: Follow-up Studies and Their Consequences*. New York: International Universities Press.

Strachey, J. (1934) The Nature of the Therapeutic Action of Psycho-Analysis. *International Journal of Psychoanalysis* 15:127–159.

Windholz, E. (1955) Problems of Termination of the Training Analysis. *Journal of the American Psychoanalytic Association* 3:641–650.

4 Three Transferences

I don't think it's been emphasized enough that from the very beginning, Freud (1912) had *two* definitions of transference. I mention this because there was a tendency to take Freud's first definition, where the transference was seen primarily as connected to internalized images of important object relations, as the only meaning of transference. We are all familiar with such interpretations. "You're viewing me now as your cruel father, waiting for you to slip up so I can criticize you." These types of interpretations are important as a means of helping the patient see how his perceptions of others can be influenced by past relationships, but it's not the only understanding Freud had about the transference.

In this same paper, Freud suggests a broader definition of transference, seeing the analytic relationship representing the stage on which the patient re-enacts his *symptoms, memories, dreams, and current experiences; that is, the transference can be a state of mind in the analysis, not only a representation of past object relations.* Freud also reminded us to treat the patient's illness as an *actual force, active at the moment, and not as an event in his past life.*

This duality of the transference as a result of a repetition of past object relations, and *a state of mind in relationship to the analyst,* is seen in this famous paragraph from *Remembering, Repeating, and Working Through* (Freud, 1914).

> For instance, the patient does not say that he remembers that he used to be defiant and critical towards his parents' authority; instead, he *behaves* in that way to the doctor. He does not remember how he came to a helpless and hopeless deadlock in his infantile sexual research; but he produces a mass of confused dreams and associations, complains that he cannot succeed in anything and asserts that he is fated never to carry through what he undertakes. He does not remember having been intensely ashamed of certain sexual activities and afraid of their being found out; but he makes it clear that he is ashamed of the treatment on which he is now embarked and tries to keep it secret from everybody. And so on.
>
> (p. 150, italics added)

DOI: 10.4324/9781032658704-6

This has come to be known, descriptively, as the enacted transference. I want to point out that what Freud described was a particular way the patient *behaved* in treatment. This is the second transference, as noted by Freud.

I believe there is a *third type of action in the transference (i.e., language action)*, which I will return to later in this chapter.

The Second Transference

In my previous work on these transferences, I have not always been clear about their differences, which I will try to correct here. What I call the *second transference* is what Freud pointed to as the manner in which the patient *behaves* in treatment. An example is the patient who readily agrees with every interpretation the analyst makes but shortly afterward shows that he disagrees with every interpretation the analyst makes. One patient who felt the need to sit up in a long analysis would look at me while he was talking and start nodding his head while giving me an imploring look. After a while I realized that without awareness, I was nodding my head in response. This need for affirmation from another couldn't be spoken about by the patient but could only be expressed in action. This wish to bask in the glow of another's eyes became understandable the further we went in the analysis. The need for mirroring was connected with shame and guilt, as Kris (1990) elaborated when describing certain narcissistic patients. These transferences that are enacted via *behavior*, once recognized, are extremely difficult to bring to the analysand's attention and often bring about a feeling in the patient of being caught in the act of something, followed by resentment toward the analyst. It often leads to an analytic impasse. This is because the behavior is driven by unconscious thoughts and feelings that can't be known at the time and can only be expressed in behavior.

Anna—The second transference

This is an example of a patient *behaving* in a certain way that is used to solve inner conflicts or have an effect on the analyst.

It is a Monday appointment and Anna[1] flies into her analytic session. Before she even lies down on the couch, Anna states, "I couldn't wait to tell you about this week-end". In a rush she begins to tell me, at great length, of the various ways her husband mistreated her. It was not told in any great distress, but more in the form of conspiratorial togetherness. It was a story I had heard many times from Anna, so her feeling that "she couldn't wait to tell me" struck me as an important indicator *of some way she was viewing the analysis and/or our relationship*. When Anna paused for a breath, I empathized with how distressing this seemed to be, and also wondered about this "couldn't wait to tell me" feeling. She cut me off saying, "Yes, Yes, but let me tell you about this other incident that happened." Anna then proceeded to tell me a lengthy story where she visited her parents, and her mother spent a long time on the phone with her sister. There were many other slights as well. I was again impressed with how propelled she was to tell me this story, again familiar, of mistreatment. My previous remarks seemed to hardly register. I felt pushed out of her narrative. Another story of a similar nature quickly followed, presented in this same breathless manner. Listening to this story I sensed an excited quality in her breathlessness. After a brief silence, I said to Anna that, again, she seemed in a *rush* to tell me what happened, so much so that it seemed difficult to register what I said. After a brief pause, Anna said, "I hate your voice". Puzzled and intrigued, I waited. She then said, "I had a sexual dream about you last night. It wasn't you in the dream, but it was a tall guy with a beard. We made love in the most tender and exciting way. When we finished, I cried. Obviously, I didn't want to tell you. It makes me so sad when I think of being loved instead of fucked. Better to go on feeling angry about being fucked than this overwhelming sadness. It's really scary. But maybe the dream indicates it's not as scary as it was."

In this example, Anna needs to keep taking actions (i.e., flying into the office, talking non-stop, interrupting me) so that she doesn't have to hear me, and then remembers her dream from the previous evening about not feeling this "overwhelming sadness".

The Third Transference

The third transference is when the patient uses words to create some feeling in the analyst and is what I've labeled as *language action*. Loewald (1975) was one of the first analysts of the modern era to discuss action in speech. He captured the ubiquity of language action in psychoanalytic treatment when he stated, "We take the patient less and less as speaking merely about himself, about his experiences and memories, and more and more as symbolizing action in speech" (p. 366). It is my understanding that language action is used to ward off anxiety; to repair a self-state; to bring about a response from the analyst that is gratifying, traumatizing, or reinforces a resistance; and to express every other human emotion or fantasy. These are the times where we have to listen to the music that accompany the words. That is, we listen to *how* the patient talks, whereas *what* she talks about is secondary. It is reminiscent of Marshal McLuhan's (1964) well-known saying, "the medium is the message". My own attempts to define language action began in 1989, and continued in 1995, 2009, and 2013. I've described the basics of why language action occurs in Chapter 1.

Hellen

Hellen is an example of a patient who uses different types of language actions to ward off feelings of self-doubt and inadequacy.

Hellen had been in analysis for a number of years. Oftentimes I felt confused when listening to her. It seemed to me there was no associative flow that would allow me to understand what she was trying to communicate. When I realized that her words were not designed to communicate, I began to focus on how she used them.

The first thing I noticed was that she would often start a sentence, interrupt herself, then go to what seemed like a different topic, and then back again to the original theme. While I can usually find meaning in such a sequence, I was more perplexed than enlightened by the themes Hellen touched on. When I pointed to the sequence of her thoughts, and how I was confused by what she said, Hannah would *explain* what she meant, rather than being able to reflect on what I said.

I also realized Hellen would always speak in an authoritative tone, mostly about external events. There was rarely a question she asked herself (e.g., "Hmm, I wonder why that came to mind?"), or a doubt she expressed about her view of things.[2] Further, her thinking was highly intellectualized and was filled with references to obscure Greek and Roman poets, the purpose of which seemed to be to show the breadth of her classical education. Often, any question I raised was experienced by her as "hurtful".

Over time, we could understand Hellen's authoritative, intellectualized approach as a defense against her low self-esteem. She could go from feeling assured and superior to feeling ugly and a nothing in an eye-blink. There was no in-between state. Her use of language that was confusing was more difficult to unravel. Eventually she was able to tell me that her parents came to the United States from a foreign country before she was born. The parents never taught her the language they grew up with, and when her parents spoke together, they would often drift into speaking their native tongue. She always felt left out of these conversations, and it infuriated her, as it touched on her feelings of being raised by an absent, critical mother. Turning passive to active, I was now the one who was confused and left out of Hannah's conversation.

Interpreting the Three Transferences

Of the three transferences, I find the second the most difficult to interpret, as it is typically first understood via the analyst's countertransference, and the behavior that leads to the countertransference is unconscious. As mentioned earlier, bringing unconscious behaviors to a patient's attention most often leads the patient to feel resentful. Further, how we translate our countertransference into *usable interpretations* by the analysand is one of the most complicated and contentious issues in psychoanalysis. For example, as I've stated (Busch, 2019), it is hard for me to see how interpretations from some post-Bionions based on the analyst's countertransference could be understood by the patient. In general, I find it necessary to try and create a good-enough atmosphere where the patient feels supported and contained before describing a countertransference feeling leading to an interpretation.

In the third transference, it is easier for the analyst to describe how the analysand is using language action based on the patient's own words. It is happening before us in the *here and now* of the session. As I've mentioned previously, because of certain qualities of the mind, the patient can primarily grasp what needs to be transformed in the *here and now*.

Finally, the ease of making the first type of transference interpretation depends on whether the interpretation is based on the analyst's countertransference or the observable here and now of the patient's words.

In Betty Joseph's (1985) ground-breaking paper on "The Total Transference", she explains her views on the importance of countertransference feelings in understanding the *enacted transferences*. Here is one example she presents that exemplifies the problem of interpreting such transferences in a way that can be integrated by the patient.

When I started to rethink my countertransference and his material, I realized that my rather gratified experience must correspond to an inner conviction on the patient's part that whatever I interpreted he was somehow all right. Whatever difficulties, even tormenting qualities in him, the work might show, there was an inner certainty that he had some very special place, that my interpretations were, as it were, 'only interpretations'. His place was assured, and he had no need to change. One could, therefore, have gone on and on making quasi-correct and not unuseful interpretations, exploring and explaining things, but if the deeper unconscious conviction remained unexamined, the whole treatment could have become falsified. This conviction of his special place and no need to change had an additional quality because it included the notion that I, the analyst, had a particular attachment to or love for him, and that for my own sake I would not wish to let him go—which I think was basic to my comfortable countertransference experience.

(p. 449)

This paper, which had a huge impact on how transference was interpreted, evades the issue of how we metabolize our countertransference reactions in a way that allows us to make an interpretation that doesn't bypass the preconscious.

How I work with my countertransference reactions can be seen below. What I would like to highlight here is the importance of clarifying the *action taking place* before offering an interpretation of the meaning of the action.

Eliot[3]

I will begin with a typical example of the transferencecountertransference dynamic with a patient who used a *combination of language action and represented associations* to express an unconscious transference dynamic. The patient, Eliot, was in his forties, very smart but a chronic underachiever. He had been underemployed since graduating from a prestigious college. He was married, blamed his wife's clinging behavior for keeping him from opportunities, and was generally angry at the world around him. A violent outburst at his wife scared him and led him to seek treatment.

Growing up, Eliot was said to have developed normally until his mother went back to work when he was two, and he reacted with a severe regression in speech and toilet training. Over time, Eliot's mother became increasingly depressed, resulting in several hospitalizations starting when he was in latency. Although he had an older sister and brother, for some time I thought he was an only child, as much of what he shared about his childhood was about being alone. In addition to depression, his mother struggled with alcoholism, resulting in angry, seemingly irrational outbursts. At the beginning of treatment, his father, a successful investment advisor, was devalued, although, as it turned out, he was the more consistent maternal presence in the home.

Eliot was in the fourth year of analysis, and it was two weeks before I was to have surgery that was going to keep me out of the office for 4–6 weeks. I wasn't in any imminent danger, but the need for the surgery came up suddenly. When I told Eliot about this several weeks before, in his characteristic manner, he said a few formal words of sympathy. Then he immediately began to talk about what had happened the previous weekend, which took up most of the session. This was his usual manner of dealing with absences, but I was struck by his non-reaction to what I'd just told him.

I felt deadened and withdrawn from what Eliot was telling me. I wondered about a projective identification or an unconscious attempt to angrily or defensively deaden me for abandoning him. However, I also realized I was narcissistically vulnerable at this time, so who was contributing what to my withdrawn and deadened state of mind was unclear. I had already informed a number of patients about the surgery and impending absence by the time I told Eliot. While some had a similar reaction to Eliot's, my feelings about their reactions were not similar to those I had with Eliot, so I wondered if there was something more than only my fragile narcissism fueling my reaction. I had to consider if there were reasons I had this reaction to Eliot more than other patients. What came to mind was surprising. Earlier in treatment, Eliot objected to my practice of charging him for missed appointments, since he "knew" he was wealthier than most patients and therefore he could take more vacations, and thus felt he was being penalized by my policy. There was little room to work with Eliot's grandiose view of himself as an "exception" at the time, and we agreed on a compromise solution for the moment. I wondered if I was still irritated with his "depriving" me of my fee. I was especially vulnerable to feeling "deprived" given that my sense of myself as an active, healthy man was challenged by this surgery. However, what was occurring in Eliot's mind was unclear to me.

As I returned to listening to the words and music of Eliot's narrative, I noticed two things. The first was a cadence to his voice, which was different. Eliot was usually a non-stop talker, and his associations were often lively. It was this libidinal investment in his thoughts and mind that led me, in the beginning, to have hope for a positive analytic outcome, in spite of his life-failures over the past 20 years. In this session I realized there were unusual pauses, and I kept feeling I was losing the connection to where he started and ended a series of thoughts. It was this loss of connection via the cadence of his speech that caught my attention as one possible factor in my countertransference withdrawal. While the obvious content interpretation of my now being the "lost" one, as a projection of Eliot's split off feelings of loss came to mind, *I first pointed to the change in the cadence of Eliot's speech, and the difficulty I was having following his thoughts.* He hadn't noticed it but could see it once I brought it to his attention. He also realized he was losing his train of thought while he was talking. Eliot's thoughts then turned to a meeting he was at where, throughout, he was highly attuned to what others were thinking of him. His preoccupation revolved around whether others were thinking he was too loud, too brash, or putting himself forward too much. As Eliot elaborated on this story, I found myself thinking of his narcissistic, depressed mother, who he felt he had to care for from childhood through most of his early adult life. When his mother locked herself in her bedroom and threatened suicide after a fight with his father, it was Eliot who was sent by the father to coax her out of her room. Throughout his life he felt he had to be what his mother wanted him to be so that she could be enlivened. For him, it was a matter of life and death. He was her self-object. It took me a while to understand that after his mother died, Eliot's lament that he couldn't keep his mother alive was a metaphor, and not simply magical thinking. Eliot also felt his mother wanted him to be a "potato", and she would call him "my little potato". For Eliot, this represented how his mother wanted him to be "silently growing" out of sight, causing no problems, except when she needed him to entertain her. In this one can also see the symbolic meaning of Eliot's mother seeing him as food or nourishment, where his presence had to feed her.

My countertransference reaction, Eliot's association to the meeting, and my associations led me to say the following:

FB: After we both notice losing the connections in what you were saying, your thoughts go to a meeting where you're worried that you're drawing too much attention to yourself. I wonder if this is similar to concerns you had when I told you about my surgery?

Eliot: I felt selfish. You were the one having surgery and my thoughts should be more about you. But I got scared. This bad thing was happening and how would I do? Then I told myself you would be fine, and I calmed down.

FB: So, reassuring yourself that I would be OK blotted out your feelings of being scared, which worried you because you felt you weren't focusing enough on me.

Eliot: (through tears) I just had another thought. When I saw you today you seemed to be holding your arm in an awkward position, as if you were in pain. As I thought that, I felt some pains in my chest.

FB: Maybe we can say you were drawn to even feel my pain.

Eliot: I remember, near the end of my mother's life, how I felt sick to my stomach all the time. (His mother died of stomach cancer.) But I felt I had to be chipper and upbeat, pretending like I didn't know the end was near. (Eliot began sobbing for several minutes.) I don't know why I keep thinking this. (He then tells an elaborate story of a very expensive trip he is planning for his wife's birthday even though it isn't at a good time for him.)

FB: Just like you felt you had to sacrifice your own worries to take care of me, you do the same with Robyn (his wife).

Eliot: When you say that I start to feel anxious. I know Robyn doesn't feel like she needs this kind of extravagant vacation, and it's the worst possible time for me. Yet I still feel like I have to do it.

As we can see, Eliot's unresponsiveness to my informing him of my impending surgery is, in fact, the result of a complex reaction. Eliot's concern for his own welfare immediately arouses anxiety over being "selfish", and his focus shifts to how he should be concerned about me. However, showing concern also seems to be threatening (i.e., as it's associated with losing himself) and the resultant compromise formation is silence, as Eliot reassures himself that I will be OK. Eliot ends up having no concern for himself or me, and the analysis goes on as if nothing has happened. This "nothing happened" is what we frequently interpret as an attack against the analyst (as I felt in my first countertransference reaction), when in this instance we can see it as an attack against the self (i.e., Eliot's worries for himself need to be discarded due to anxiety) and, as we shall see, a protection of the object.

Listening to Eliot's associations, we hear that he is afraid others are seeing him as self-centered. When I'm able to connect this concern with his unresponsiveness, Eliot is able to feel the pain he first ignored. However, it is another's pain. It is what he imagines as my pain, just as he was only able to feel his mother's pain as she was dying. He cannot easily feel his own pain, as it is frightening and dangerous. "Selfish" is the word he uses to describe being "scared" when I tell him of my operation. He must turn his attention to the object and pretend like nothing happened, or his tenuous connection to the object will be shattered.

Eliot's thoughts then lead us to see another meaning in his "not noticing", that is, caring for the object. Thus, he needs to "not notice" when his mother is dying, just like he didn't notice when his mother was hospitalized, and like he didn't notice his mother's narcissistic self-involvement or angry tirades, and, most importantly, his own reactions to any of this. His associations lead him to how he is driven to care for his wife, even recognizing that it has little to do with her. In Eliot's mind, caring for a woman is to literally keep her alive, and thus to feel enlivened himself. This was his job in life—to keep his mother alive. "Not noticing" became one way of doing this, and thus its manifestation in the transference–countertransference when I tell him of my impending surgery.

In working with my countertransference reaction, I first pointed to what Eliot is doing with his speech (i.e., losing connections), rather than interpreting the meaning or content of projecting his feeling of loss (e.g., "Your way of talking leaves me feeling a loss of connection. I wonder if in this way I'm the one who feels the loss rather than you"). Instead, I point to what is potentially most observable within the transference–countertransference dynamic. This leaves it up to Eliot to see which part, if any, he is able to deal with during this complicated time in the treatment. As happens with more neurotically organized patients, an association comes to mind that allows for a greater understanding of one aspect of Eliot's reaction to my surgery and lengthy absence.

One can see in this example the complexity of understanding transference reactions, and the importance of having in mind the different transferences. Initially we learn of Eliot's concern of being viewed as selfish, leading to an action (not bringing up his fears), followed by his using language action (i.e., a different cadence to his speech which I find confusing); when clarified, an association comes to mind of his mother's illness, and his psychosomatic reaction at the time, and is repeated in the session. Thus, in this one vignette, we can see the three different types of transferences shown in succession, which lead to different reactions (i.e., action and language action leading to a *countertransference reaction*, which, once understood, leads to a *clarification*, which in turn brings about a series of associations that leads to an *interpretation*.) Recognizing these different transferences can lead to subtlety in technique in contrast to viewing everything the patient says as a reference to the analyst.

Notes

1   Previously appeared in *Creating a Psychoanalytic Mind*.
2   This patient was also someone who couldn't experience "pleasant passivity" as Michael Fain described it, and as was elaborated on by Aisenstein (2022).
3   Previously presented in Busch (2013).

References

Aisenstein, M. (2022) *Desire, Pain and Thought*. London: Routledge.

Busch, F. (2009) 'Can You Push a Camel through the Eye of a Needle?' Reflections on how the Unconscious Speaks to us and its Clinical Implications. *International Journal of Psychoanalysis* 90:53–68.

Busch, F. (2013) *Creating a Psychoanalytic Mind*. London: Routledge.

Busch, F. (2019) *The Analyst's Reveries*. London: Routledge.

Freud, S. (1912) The Dynamics of Transference. The Standard Edition of the Complete Psychological Works of Sigmund Freud 12:97–108

Freud, S. (1914) Remembering, repeating, and working through. The Standard Edition of the Complete Psychological Works of Sigmund Freud 14:145–156.

Joseph, B. (1985) Transference: The Total Situation. *International Journal of Psychoanalysis* 66:447–454.

Kris, A.O. (1990) The Analyst's Stance and the Method of Free Association. *Psychoanalytic Study of the Child* 45:25–41.

Loewald, H.W. (1975) Psychoanalysis as an Art and the Fantasy Character of the Psychoanalytic Situation. *Journal of the American Psychoanalytic Association* 23: 277–299.

McLuhan, Marshall (1964) *Understanding Media: The Extensions of Man*. Cambridge, MA: MIT Press.

5 Ethical Countertransference

Heimann's (1950) ground-breaking paper on countertransference posited that the analyst's unbidden reveries, thoughts, feelings, and fantasies could be understood as his/her unconscious resonating with the patient's unconscious. It potentially brought a new dimension to the analyst's way of understanding countertransference, while the predominant position at the time was expressed by Annie Reich (1951) when she stated one year later:

> Counter-transference thus comprises the effects of the analyst's own unconscious needs and conflicts on his understanding or technique. In such cases the patient represents for the analyst an object of the past on to whom past feelings and wishes are projected, just as it happens in the patient's transference situation with the analyst.
>
> (p. 26)

Thus, Heimann brought out of the shadows what analysts had been struggling to guiltily hide for many years.

The developments since then have been covered extensively by Jacobs (1999), Spillius and O'Shaughnessy (2012), Diamond (2014), and many others. We find that over the last 70 years, a wide variety of views grew as to how countertransference is understood and used clinically by analysts. On one side of the continuum are those who basically follow Heimann's central thesis. On the other side, there are those analysts who view countertransference reactions as a complex psychic phenomenon with no single cause. An example of those who strictly follow Heimann is Ogden (1997), who states,

> As personal and private as our reveries feel to us, it is misleading to view them as "our" personal creations, since reverie is at the same time an aspect of a jointly (but asymmetrically) created unconscious intersubjective constructions that I have termed the intersubjective analytic third.
>
> (p. 569)

DOI: 10.4324/9781032658704-7

In 2006, Pine, while generally open to the importance of the mutual influence of the two parties in the analytic situation, presciently suggested that:

> With the current flood of attention to transference, enactment, role-responsiveness, positive use of countertransference, and the inevitability of mutual two-way influences in the analytic session, there is a danger that the significance of the other stages, the ones we did quite well with before we had all these new ones, will be forgotten.
>
> (pp. 474–475)

In an earlier paper (2001), Pine described the dangers of using countertransference as an unerring guide to the patient's unconscious.

> Surely, we have all seen instances, in supervision or in writings, where a therapist or analyst took something personal to be about the patient—while the listener or reader is, to say the least, not convinced. Speaking for myself, I have unquestionably (to me, by my standards of evidence) found powerful instances where I am thus informed about the patient. *On the other hand, my reveries or distracted thoughts often seem to me to be more about me than the patient.* I say that because I note that they can occur indiscriminately with anyone, they can occur when I am alone, and they are recognizably reflective of what I know about myself.
>
> (pp. 907–908, italics added)

Tuch (2015), amongst many others, echoed Pine's position when he states, "Current trends that overemphasize the two-person psychological perspective contribute to our forgetting that we all bring our own psychologies—our *separable subjectivities*—to the consulting room, independent of the analytic third that is constituted once the process gets underway" (p. 385). Or, as Cassorla (2013) succinctly put it, "It is important to note that even though the analyst's dream is a dream for two, *it is a dream of his or her own*" (p. 204, italics added). My purpose in this chapter is to question whether, from these widely different views, we can find an ethically viable use of the countertransference. I put it this way as some current views of countertransference seem not congruent with generally agreed upon psychoanalytic principles.

Re-Reading Heimann and Racker

In a close reading of these two authors, whom most psychoanalysts consider the forerunners of an expanded view of countertransference, there are *warnings* against a wholesale acceptance of the view that the

analyst's countertransference derives only from an unconscious understanding of the analysand's unconscious transference. I will briefly
present their main viewpoints before turning to their cautions.

Compared to its length (three pages), Heimann's (1950) paper had
an outsized influence. Her thesis was stated in the following way:

> Our basic assumption is that the analyst's unconscious understands
> that of his patient. This rapport on the deep level comes to the sur-
> face in the form of feelings which the analyst notices in response to
> his patient, in his counter-transference. This is the most dynamic
> way in which his patient's voice reaches him.
>
> (p. 82)

Racker (1953, 1957) published two important papers on countertransference, with his first paper being presented to the Argentine
Psychoanalytic Society 2 years before Heimann's paper appeared in
print. In his second paper, he says he agrees with Heimann, and while
still seeing countertransference as central to the analyst's work with
patients, he defined a more specific basis for countertransference than
Heimann did. His 1957 views revolve around two specific identifications, *concordant* and *complementary*. As LaFarge (2007) described
concordant identifications:

> the analyst identifies himself with the patient by aligning his own
> mind with the patient's—his ego with the patient's ego, his super-
> ego with the patient's superego, and his id with the patient's id. In
> this mode, the patient's conflicts come alive through their resonance
> with analogous conflicts in the analyst. This kind of identification
> corresponds to what people ordinarily call *empathy*, and the ana-
> lyst subjectively feels that he understands his patient.
>
> (p. 800)

In complementary identifications, the analyst identifies himself with
the patient's internal structures (e.g., superego), or internal objects.
This is the noisier countertransference sometimes leading to the analyst's enactments, or, as LaFarge put it, "when the analyst feels something *toward* his patient rather than feeling *with* him" (p. 80).

In spite of the emphasis on countertransference as an unconscious
understanding, both authors *express a caution that has tended to
be overlooked.* This caution refers to the analyst's assumption that
his unconscious countertransference is *perfectly aligned with the
patient's unconscious.* While for much of her paper Heimann emphasizes this alignment, there is a brief passage where she acknowledges
that the analyst must consider his *personal reactions*, which needs
to be analyzed. After describing how the analyst needs to use his

emotional response to understand his patient's unconscious, she states, "*At the same time he will find ample stimulus for taking himself to task again and again and for continuing the analysis of his own problems*" (p. 83, italics added). This briefly resonates with her earlier statement that "The approach to the counter-transference which I have presented is not without danger. It does not represent a screen for the analyst's shortcomings" (p. 83). Thus, while Heimann generally takes the position that the analyst's "unconscious perception of the patient's unconscious is more acute and in advance of his conscious conception of the situation" (p. 82), she notes briefly that he needs to be alert to the idiosyncrasies and distorting effects of his own unconscious. In a 1956 paper, Heimann was even more forceful in reminding us that countertransference could be a result of the analyst's own problems and need to be analyzed. In fact, O'Shaughnessy (2012) reminds us that Heimann, in writing about projective identification, eventually concluded that it "occurs as a countertransference phenomenon when the analyst fails in his perceptive functions" (ibid., p. 156).

In Racker's (1953) first paper, he is quite specific in warning the analyst to be wary of considering all his countertransference reactions as concordant. He points out that "the counter-transference may help, distort, or hinder the *perception* of the unconscious processes" (p. 313). Or again, the analyst's "*perception may be correct, but the percept may provoke neurotic reactions which impair his interpretive capacity*" (p. 313). Even after analysis:

> part of his libido remains fixated in phantasy—to the introjected objects—and so apt to be transferred. Part of his psychic conflicts remain unsolved and strive after a solution by means of relations with external objects. His profession, too, and his resulting social and financial situation are subject to the transference of central inner situations.
>
> (p. 313)

Thus, neither Heimann nor Racker believe *the analyst should entirely forgo responsibility for his countertransference thoughts, feelings, or reveries.* In ignoring these early warnings, some analysts end up on a slippery slope towards believing in an *empathic unconscious,* an oxymoron given that since its discovery the preponderance of analysts view the unconscious as a cauldron of irrationality and selfishness, with barely represented forces striving for gratification. Thus, given what we know about unconscious functioning, the analyst's *ethically responsible position when experiencing a countertransference would seem to be to consult his own mind before assigning his reaction to an attunement with the patient's unconscious.*

A Proposal for an Ethically Sound Countertransference Position

Diamond (2014) raised the issue of an ethical transgression when the analyst uses his mental experiences in the extreme, forgetting about the patient's psychology. I suggest the same question needs to be asked when *the analyst considers his multitudinous unconscious or even pre-conscious countertransference reactions are viewed as solely, or even predominantly, a reflection of the patient's unconscious.* There are two basic ideas that makes such a claim unlikely. First of all, given that the unconscious is unknowable, it would take considerable self-analytic work for an unconscious reaction to become preconsciously available and useable by the analyst. Thus, some essential transformation would have to take place, just as it would for the patient's unconscious to be changed from a barely formed idea to a symbolic representation. Secondly, as Racker (1953) emphasized, there is no such thing as the perfectly analyzed analyst. This is why the idea of an analyst's unconscious, unfettered by personal idiosyncrasies, intuiting the patient's unconscious in some pure form, seems like a fiction.

Therefore, I propose that an *ethical countertransference position* necessitates considerable self-analytic work in sorting through the innumerable possibilities when experiencing a countertransference reaction. What is this self-analytic work I refer to? I believe with Barratt (2017) that any self-analytic inquiry begins with the analyst's associations. As Barratt expressed it:

> only free-association methodically opens the discourse of self-consciousness (the representations available to reflective awareness) to the voicing of the repressed. The method is key to Freud's original-ity and the *sine qua non* of any genuinely psychoanalytic process. Clinical procedures which do not prioritize a steadfast and ongoing commitment to this method ... (limit the) capacity to divulge the power of unconscious processes.
>
> (p. 39, parenthesis added)

However, it isn't only the analyst's capacity to freely associate that leads to self-analysis; it requires that we observe, reflect, and play with our associations in a way that leads to self-inquiry. Self-inquiry is a term introduced by Gardner (1983) as a place in the mind where the capacity to play with ideas as a basis for understanding exists. It is a place where newly created ideas can be freely explored, a place for curious musings. It is akin to what Viderman (1974) described as an *analytic space*, an imaginary place, the construction of which develops in analysis so that there is a place where the analytic process is going to find all its force and explore all its possibilities. It requires the analyst to take the time to see what *reverberates* from his/her initial reaction as Birksted-Breen (2009, 2012) captured it. As expressed by Diamond (2014), this *mind use* by the analyst is a "constant, essential factor in the complex process of therapeutic action" (p. 533).

It isn't a fool-proof system, as there will be times when, for a variety of reasons, we may miss the signs of a personal countertransference reaction. *However, as analysts, it is the main tool we have to understand ourselves, just as it is for our patients.*

It is also worth noting that there is no such thing as *a* countertransference; rather there are *levels* of countertransference. Thus, the analyst's brief fantasy while a patient is talking is already an occurrence in symbolic form, while a psychosomatic reaction is without representation. The fantasy is likely more easily analyzed than the psychosomatic reaction.

Mr. B

In this session, I feel an urge toward what could have been a countertransference enactment. Subsequently, my own associations and the patient's helped me understand what this push to enact was about and opened an important dimension of the treatment.

Mr. B was talking about an interaction with his mother, the kind of interaction we had analyzed many times before. At these times he picked up what he felt was a subtle hostility on her part, which he pushed away, replacing it with an idealized view of her. His reaction seemed like what Fairbairn (1952) described as a "moral defense", where the good object is held on to for a desperate sense of security, and the child introjects the view of himself as the bad object. Mr. B had made good progress, and no longer had to view himself as the bad object to protect his sense of security. However, in reporting the current conversation, it seemed like he'd forgotten everything we'd talked about, and the old dynamic was repeated. Instead of how I might usually think of this as a temporary regression to deal with something stirred up in the interaction, I found myself irritated. I wondered about a projective identification, but nothing came to mind. Shortly afterwards, about a minute before the end of the session, Mr. B's associations led me to think I understood something new about the multiple meanings of his characterological depression. I felt an *urge* to tell Mr. B what I thought. It was this *driven* quality that caught my attention and gave me pause. If what I was thinking had any validity, it would be important to give Mr. B the space to react to my interpretation, and for me to follow the chain of associations that ensued. I didn't say anything, and the session ended.

A few minutes after Mr. B left the session, I felt sad. My thoughts immediately went to the unspoken interpretation, and then to my surprise I thought of Andre Green's (1986) concept of the "dead mother". This thought was followed by my remembering a statement a supervisor of mine once made that "all analysts are trying to cure their depressed mothers". This made a lot of sense to me given my own history, and I had been impressed in talking personally with other analysts over many years how this was also the case for them. Indeed, what I felt as an urge to say at the end of the session had to do with Mr. B's identification with the depressed side of his manic-depressed mother. In returning to my feelings of sadness after the session with Mr. B, I wondered if the pressure I felt to interpret was based on a fantasy of a missed opportunity to say something that would miraculously lead him out of his depression. In this fantasy I would have finally cured my depressed mother-patient.

At this point I had forgotten about my feelings of irritation, but something was nagging at me during the day. Later on, I did remember my irritation and wondered how it fit with my associations, and the urge to act at the end of the session. These rescue fantasies to cure a mother now seemed like a defense against what I felt was projected, that is, Mr. B's irritation with his mother. Did I feel I had to protect myself and Mr. B against this anger towards a mother? This is where I was before the next session. My associations left me with many questions as to the meaning of my almost enactment.

In the following session, Mr. B's initial affect was blunted, and he talked about a familiar characterological pattern, without awareness, of how he unconsciously gets people to pin him down and then resents it. I felt this was also being enacted in the session in that Mr. B would make an interesting but ambiguous reference to something, and I would find myself wanting to question him in a way that would "pin him down". I wondered if this had enlivened Mr. B's mother, as the main connection she seemed to have with him was via criticizing him. I remembered, then, that although I considered Mr. B a very competent person, I would often have questions in my mind about his business decisions. At these times I would find myself taking on the role of the knowledgeable advisor, although I knew nothing about his area of expertise. I became aware of how I seemed to be enacting the role of his "know it all" mother, but I felt there was more I wasn't grasping.

Towards the middle of the session, Mr. B, in a livelier fashion, found himself surprised at how un-lively he seemed. He contrasted it with how he felt after leaving the previous session, when he felt incredibly joyful, hopeful, and full of energy. This surprised and intrigued me given my own reaction. He went on to say that for the first time in a long time, what he wanted and needed to do seemed less effortful. He was able to see many things we had talked about in the past. His first association after this was to Icarus. Icarus' plight had come up from time to time in the past, especially in dreams. However, as Mr. B began to talk about this, his affect became desultory. I brought this to his attention, suggesting that something had just happened to change how he seemed to feel. His thoughts turned to the previous day when he was given a leadership role over an older man in his firm. After a brief moment of feeling joyful, he felt anxious, and felt the need to ask this man for help on an upcoming project.

I wondered with him if we could understand his less lively self as a cautionary tale to protect us both. I was thinking of his conflictual reaction to the wish to fly higher than me, and the *danger* this seemed to bring about for him (i.e., think Icarus). His thoughts went to his concern (previously discussed) of spinning out of control, getting angry, and being destructive. While Mr. B's fear of being destructive if he felt too excited had come up before, it seemed there was something immediate he was defending against in the transference–countertransference, and that was his wish/fear of flying higher than me and in his mind, destroying me. After all, it was immediately after his spontaneous association to Icarus and his sense that this was meaningful, both of which seemed like the beginning capacity to *use his own psychoanalytic mind* (Busch, 2013), that his desultory mood began. I found myself formulating an interpretation of the above, when I realized how close we were to the end of the session, leading me, again, to not say anything. In contrast to the previous session, I felt pleased at the end of the session that Mr. B was finding *his* way, like a benevolent father would feel. This also caught my attention. He returned the following session in a desultory mood but became lively again as the session progressed.

Reflections

I think this vignette shows something of the complex meanings when we feel driven to interpret by our own countertransference. At these times, it raises a question: "Who we are trying to cure?" With Mr. B, the push to say something seemed an attempt, in part, to cure my internalized depressed mother. However, the emergence of Mr. B's own self-analytic capacities (including his capacity to freely associate), and the Icarus fears that came immediately afterward, allowed me to consider an entirely different way of thinking about what had happened. My urge to say something at the end of the session, that in my own mind would be *crucial* to his understanding, now seemed to me to be like being an overly helpful paternal figure, masking (and enacting) my competitiveness, by feeling it was only *my* understanding that could help him. At some level, I must have realized he was flying high in the session, and there was no need for me to say anything. His capacity to do this again in the following session was a further indication of Mr. B's burgeoning analytic mind. It then seemed possible that my sadness was associated with a father's realization that his son was indicating his readiness to start moving out on his own, mixed in with a defense over my own wish to be the one with all the expertise. Thus, my urge to say something to Mr. B seems to have been driven by forces within me to cure a number of issues for myself. If I had spoken at the end of the session, I think it would have unconsciously pulled Mr. B back from his feelings of soaring and made it more difficult to associate to his related fears.

This vignette shows the complexities of our work, especially when countertransference is involved. My initial associations led me to think of my urge to say something as a partially neurotically induced need to cure a depressed mother. However, Mr. B's associations led to other possibilities regarding fathers and sons, competition, and a need to claim my superior position. Listening to my associations and the reverberations from Mr. B's session led me to be alert to two possible countertransference reactions I was having to Mr. B. It is this type of self-analytic work that seems necessary to gain some grasp on our unconscious participation in clinical work and offers the best protection we have against mixing up our unconscious with the patient's. I believe it is the best we can do to approach an ethical way of dealing with our countertransference.

Forms of Understanding Countertransference

In this section, I will discuss varying ways of conceiving and dealing with countertransference reactions.

Projective Identification

This complex, highly debated defense mechanism was never fully accepted by Klein, as she didn't believe that countertransference could be used as useful information about the patient (Spillius, 1992). As Hinz (2012) noted, she:

> had doubts about its usefulness and was afraid it would be misused as an alibi for the analyst's own insufficiencies because he might downplay the complexities of the analytic relationship and blame his own emotional reaction on the patient without working on them, integrating and convert them further reflexively.
>
> (p. 192)

My concerns about a static use of the concept mirror that of Klein.

Amongst certain analysts, there is a tendency to believe that whatever they are feeling is the result of projective identification (e.g., Director, 2009; Waska, 2016). However, there are those like Michael

Feldman (2012), who, in his typically lucid description of the topic, warns against such an approach. He points to the analyst's difficulty in being aware of defensively employed, gratifying fantasies, that preclude the unconscious anxieties evoked by the patient's projections to emerge. This can include a belief in one's comfortable, dispassionate involvement. He describes how when under the pressure of a projective identification the analyst may enact complex object relationships to reassure them both, or, faced with an unacceptable version of himself, he may attack the patient or terminate treatment. He is sympathetic to the difficulty and pain "for the analyst to recognize the subtle enactments he is inevitably drawn into by the patient, and to find understanding outside the confines unconsciously demanded by the patient" (p. 125). The patient's archaic unconscious object relationships inevitably touch on the analyst's unresolved conflicts, and enactments ensue to gratify a mutual need or defend against it. "The analyst's temporary and partial recovery of his capacity for reflective thought rather than action is crucial for the survival of his analytic role" (p. 131).

I would like to return now to an analysis described by Brown (2015), previously mentioned in Chapter 1. I pointed out that one can see how the *assumption* of a feeling experienced by the analyst as a projective identification can lead to losing touch with the patient, and that this can be found again when, after some reflection, the analyst becomes aware of an enactment due to feelings stirred up within him. I will use Brown's material as an example of how an assumption of the analyst's feelings as a projective identification, *without further associations*, can lead one to solipsistic thinking, which can be reversed when the analyst is able to *reflect* on what is occurring in his own mind. It is to Brown's credit that it only took a few sessions before realizing he was engaged in an enactment. As Feldman noted, this type of unconscious enactment is one of the most difficult for all analysts to recognize.

To remind the reader, in the third year of treatment, Brown's patient suddenly announces he is terminating the treatment at the end of the session and does so. I will repeat what I reported earlier, before showing how Brown recovering his analytic mind leads him to a different understanding.

Mr. R's sudden decisions to immediately end the analysis, though clearly related to fears of dependency and homoerotic anxieties, occurred without any apparent warning: he simply and calmly said he was not returning and thanked me for my help. The manner in which he abruptly ended our work understandably left me feeling blindsided, weak, and helpless. As I reflected on Mr. R's mode of ending, it seemed clear that his feelings of "gayness" and dependency had been projected into me and had now become my burden with which to struggle, leaving me feeling weakened and impotent.

(pp. 852–853)

While most analysts would feel blindsided by such a sudden termination, it's not clear or explained why the patient's "gayness" and dependency, if projected into Brown, would make him feel "weakened and impotent". It seems to be a use of a plugged-in theory to explain an uncomfortable feeling, and helps the analyst avoid the anxiety of further exploration. I would think that in such a situation one might also be thinking about whether one had misunderstood something that led the patient to need to leave to protect against any number of painful psychic feelings.

When the patient returns to treatment, Brown puts his feelings back into him when he says:

After his return, I brought up his leaving suddenly as a means by which he got rid of feeling weak and gay, and instead sought to evoke those emotions in me—i.e., 'giving' them to me as my problem to handle.

(pp. 852–853)

The patient superficially agreed with this intervention, but it seemed to have no effect upon him according to Brown.

Here Brown, still unable to advance his reflections, remains under the belief that this is all projective identification, and then shoves it back into the patient, a technique that I think otherwise Brown would see as not particularly helpful. It seems understandable that this interpretation would have little effect. If this indeed was a major defense his patient used, how can we think that by just telling the patient this is the case, he would agree? Defenses are there because the patient is terrified of certain feelings, which Brown well knows. So, this seems to be a defensive enactment on Brown's part.

After what Brown describes as a three-month period of working well together, the patient suddenly terminates again. Brown describes how:

The attack on me as analyst was expressed by the forceful projective identification of his feelings of weakness and dependency into me, perhaps to show me the true force of these emotions to which I may not have been adequately receptive.

(p. 853)

Again, here, Brown seems to assume that *his* feelings are the result of the patient's projection. However, the danger in such a position can be seen when, later on, Brown senses there is a collusive enactment occurring in the sessions when he says:

> But it seems that deeper terrors of loss, shared by the two of us in the context of our own histories and unconsciously sensed as too unbearable for the analytic process, were projected into the analytic setting, and thereby rendered nonprocess, awaiting expression at some future point.
>
> (p. 854)

At a later time, he tells us that he felt he was over-interpreting the patient's fears of dependency and feeling abandoned because of his (i.e., Brown's) upcoming vacation. He then says, "On reflection, I was attempting to treat *my* anxiety of loss, which was likely magnified by Mr. R's projection into me of his similar fears" (p. 854).

Here we appear to be seeing Brown doing the difficult work of recognizing his role in an interpretive perspective. It seems to me this reflective process is the key to the analyst not using projective identification as a defense against exploration of his own mind. It would have been helpful to know how Brown used his analytic mind to recognize this view of a deeper terror shared by patient and analyst. It seems to me this analytic process is basic to an understanding of how the analyst comes to what he believes is an insight.

It is several pages later, almost as an afterthought, that Brown mentions:

> Fears of loss were already alive and powerful in me (my elderly father's health was fading at the time), but I failed to reflect sufficiently on my experience to realize the massive projective identification that was also in operation; thus, the analytic process had been overtaken by my fears of an actual loss and had ceased to be a field of dreams.
>
> (p. 857)

Brown's insight demonstrates the type of problem that led Klein to be wary of in the overuse of projective identification. However, Brown recapturing his capacity to stand back and understand that a more complicated countertransference reaction was being enacted speaks to what I consider an ethical countertransference position.

Relational Unconscious

Most analysts would agree with Pine (2011) that the mind is both "internally driven and relationally responsive" (p. 825). However, with the introduction of the concept of the *relational unconscious, the individual mind is taken out of the equation, and* it is proposed that countertransference reactions need to be considered *a creation of the dyad.* Instead of offering this idea as an *addition* to psychoanalytic understanding, it is presented as a *replacement* for our previous, more cautious ideas, *making irrelevant the role of our individual psyches in countertransference occurrences.*

The term "relational unconscious", which first appeared in the literature in a paper by Ahumada (1991), became part of the relational perspective after a paper by Davies (1996), and was most fully articulated by Gerson (2004). To highlight Gerson's view, it might be useful to consider a brief memory he presents of his work with a patient many years before. In this example the patient is stuck in deciding on what to do next in his professional life, and he has an association to the Bishop Berkeley conundrum presented in basic philosophy courses: "if a tree falls in the forest and no one is there to hear it, does it still make a sound?" The patient says that in order for him to know if he heard it, there would have to be another person there to ask if he heard it too. Rather than seeing this as a difficulty the patient may have in trusting his senses and knowing his own mind, Gerson views it as an example of the *communal basis of knowledge.* He goes on to state:

> The relational unconscious, as a jointly constructed process maintained by each individual in the relation, is not simply a projection of one person's unconscious self and object representations and interactional schemas onto the other, nor is it constituted by a series of such reciprocal projections and introjections between two people. Rather, as used here, the relational unconscious is the unrecognized bond that wraps each relationship, infusing the expression and constriction of each partner's subjectivity and individual unconscious within that particular relation.
>
> (p. 72)

This view is based upon the premise that:

> the organization of meaning in one mind is always embedded in processes of reciprocal influence with other minds ... The emphasis here is that the maintenance, transformation, and/or creation of organizations of meaning in one person rely on an active engagement with others (internally and/or externally) for realization.
>
> (ibid., p. 68)

From this perspective, the individual unconscious awaits elaboration in the experience with another. There is no individual mind able to reflect upon itself.

Gerson uses a clinical example from Jacobs (2001), where an impasse developed. As reported by Jacobs:

> My father's sudden illness, and my reaction to it, had the effect of disrupting this work. As I mentioned, F [the patient] retreated in the face of what he perceived as signs of disability in his analyst. Since I did not understand and therefore could not interpret the underlying fantasies that led to his withdrawal, progress in the analysis essentially came to a halt. Indirectly, however, through associations that contained references to ill, disturbed, or otherwise nonfunctioning physicians, teachers, or other authority figures, F expressed the anxious concerns that, consciously, he had managed to keep at bay. For reasons of my own, I did not pick up these messages. To do so would have been to confront my own behavior, to explore its meaning, and to come in touch with the conflictual issues concerning my father, parallel to those F was struggling with, that I, too, wished to avoid.
>
> (Jacobs, 2001, p. 16)

In Gerson's understanding, this is an example of what he calls an *intersubjective resistance* that is part of an unconscious figuration in the dyad, which goes beyond an individual resistance.

To look deeper into Jacobs' (2001) paper, he describes his work with this young man (F), whose progress in life stopped after seeing the deterioration of his father's capacities and eventual death. The treatment seemed to be going well until around 18 months, when any further advancement came to a halt. It was only after Jacobs was able to reflect on what was going on in the treatment, and *could allow himself to have associations,* that he understood what was happening. While it becomes clear that Jacobs was unconsciously enacting something with the patient, and the patient was unconsciously responding to it, *understanding came first from Jacobs' own mind, not in dyadic knowing.*

Jacobs' awareness begins when he considers that his patient's sudden obsessive focus on the realities of his relationship with his girlfriend was part of something that happened in his and F's relationship that he hadn't been able to see at the time. He realized that his patient had been making indirect comments on Jacobs' appearance. In the session that set Jacobs to thinking, the patient mentioned an analyst who went around town in odd outfits. After the session, Jacobs realized, to his surprise, that he had dressed that morning in mismatched pants and jacket.

Jacobs self-analysis began with his thoughts on:

> how foolish I must have looked, and how disorganized. Then the image of a character in a Samuel Beckett play came to mind. This

figure, aptly named Krapp, is a confused, disheveled, and demented individual on the verge of senility. Reflecting on these associations to an old man suffering from organic brain disease, I realized that they pointed to certain aspects of my behavior that I had not wanted to acknowledge; to a change in myself, in fact, which I had sought to ignore. And this change, this alteration, I recognized, was related not only to the error that I had made, but to much that had been happening in F's treatment.

(pp. 13–14)

Jacobs then tells us that some months earlier, his father had suffered a stroke that had left him partially paralyzed and suffering from some cognitive and expressive defects. Most importantly for the treatment, his father became careless about how he looked.

A man who, all his life, took pains to be well groomed and smartly dressed, now he seemed indifferent to the way that he looked. Often unkempt, he would walk around the house in an ill-fitting bathrobe or in clothes seemingly chosen at random from a dresser drawer.

Jacobs also mentions that in the time after his father's illness, he (Jacobs) began to make mistakes (e.g., miscalculated bills, forgot to tell patients of upcoming vacations, etc.), indicating cognitive decline like his father and his patient's father. From his side, Jacobs realized that he had tried to blame these errors on external factors, to avoid opening up old, painful feelings he could not confront at the time. The patient had noted these errors and immediately linked them with his own father's decline, but tried to banish these thoughts from awareness. "While this effort at suppression helped keep F's anxiety in check, it led to an unconscious holding back. Whereas, before, F was eager to be involved with me as a new father, now he withdrew and was careful to maintain a safe distance" (p. 14).

In summary, we see how Jacobs, after an enactment, *consults his own mind*, and realizes he's unconsciously been identifying with his disabled father. In this way he is able to listen again to his patient's concerns about his seeming cognitive decline, which had terrified the patient because of his personal history. While Gerson sees all this as a result of a dyadically determined resistance, it is only after Jacob's father becomes ill that he starts to evidence the behavior indicative of his unconscious identification with his father. Jacobs work seems an excellent example of an ethical manner of dealing with counter-transference. His mismatched outfit leads him to associate with the character in Samuel Beckett's play *Krapp's Last Tape*, which leads him to think of his father's cognitive decline, bringing him to realize his unconscious identification with his father, and how this prevented him from understanding the impasse that developed, that is, F's fear that Jacobs was becoming disabled like F's own father.

Ogden and Ferro

Ogden and Ferro (in his later writings) proposed the view that all analyses, and thus all countertransference reactions, are entirely co-constructed (Busch, 2019). It is a view similar to those who believe in a relational unconscious. With Ferro's (2006) belief in the powers of the *field*, he sees how the analyst's responsibility for the significance of his role in a countertransference reaction becomes increasingly irrelevant. "In the analytic field the 'subjective fields' of each participant flow together, giving rise to a new entity that is much more the sum of its predecessors" (Ferro and Basile, 2009, p. 13).

As I've reported previously, even though Ogden reports countertransference reactions that seem like primitive, unrepresented states (unpleasant somatic reactions, feelings of claustrophobia, etc.), and murderous reactions to patients, he takes no personal ownership. Instead, they are seen as co-constructed and not analyzed further.

> I do not conceive of the analytic interaction in terms of the analyst's bringing pre-existing sensitivities to the analytic relationship that are "called into play" (like keys on a piano being stuck) by the patient's projections or projective identifications. Rather I conceive of the analytic process as involving the creation of *unconscious intersubjective events* that have never previously existed in the affective life of either analyst or analysand.
>
> (Ogden, 1997, p. 589, italics added)

In short, both these authors believe that their countertransference reactions are a third entity outside of their personal contribution. Thus, in this co-constructed paradigm, we don't hear about the "co" part of the co-construction.

Concluding Thoughts

The clinical complexity involved in understanding co-created countertransferences was recognized early. However, over the years, the notion of a co-created countertransference became simplified, so that some psychoanalysts came to believe that one's unresolved unconscious issues no longer needed to be considered part of the countertransference equation. The dangers of such a position have been articulated by Feldman and others. This has led me to articulate what I consider an *ethical* approach to our countertransference, based on the analyst's self-analytic process in "reverberation time" (Birksted-Breen, 2012).

Some might say the analyst's spontaneous reaction would be lost in this way, but the patient's unconscious doesn't go away. Further, as Ahumada (1998) wrote in response to an article championing the analyst spontaneous reactions:

the basic matter here is whether, in what concerns the analyst's role, the spontaneity of "subject-to-subject impact" can be allowed to overshoot the need for a handling of the setting, and then pass on to play the inspirational role of the master, as Ferenczi tried to do in the final, "mutual analysis" period of his life, or whether we should better stick to keeping the analyst's spontaneity in the humbler role of handmaiden to the method.

(p. 943)

References

Ahumada, J.L. (1991) Logical Types and Ostensive Insight. *International Journal of Psychoanalysis* 72:683–691.

Ahumada, J.L. (1998) Psychic Deadness. By Michael Eigen. *Journal of the American Psychoanalytic Association* 46(3):940–943.

Birksted-Breen, D. (2009) Reverberation Time, Dreaming and the Capacity to Dream. *International Journal of Psychoanalysis* 90:35–51.

Birksted-Breen, D. (2012) Taking Time: The Tempo of Psychoanalysis. *International Journal of Psychoanalysis* 93(4):819–835.

Barratt, B.B. (2017) Opening to the Otherwise: The Discipline of Listening and the Necessity of Free-Association for Psychoanalytic Praxis. *International Journal of Psychoanalysis* 98(1):39–53.

Brown, L.J. (2015) Ruptures in the Analytic Setting and Disturbances in the Transformational Field of Dreams. *Psychoanalytic Quarterly* 84(4):841–865.

Busch, F. (2013) *Creating a Psychoanalytic Mind*. London: Routledge.

Busch, F. (2019) *The Analyst's Reveries: An Exploration of Bion's Enigmatic Concept*. London: Routledge.

Cassorla, R. (2013) In Search of Symbolization. In Levine, H., Reed, G. and Scarfone, D. (Eds.), *Unrepresented State sand the Construction of Meaning*. London: Routledge.

Davies, J.M. (1996) Linking the "Pre-Analytic" with the Postclassical: *Contemporary Psychoanalysis* 32:553–576.

Diamond, M.J. (2014) Analytic Mind Use and Interpsychic Communication: Driving Force in Analytic Technique, Pathway to Unconscious Mental Life. *Psychoanalytic Quarterly* 83(3):525–563.

Director, L. (2009) The Enlivening Object. *Contemporary Psychoanalysis* 45(1):120–141.

Fairbairn, W.D. (1952) *Psychoanalytic Studies of the Personality*, 1–297. London: Tavistock.

Feldman, M. (2012) Projective Identification: The Analyst's Involvement. In Spillius, E. and O'Shaughnessy, E. (eds.), *Projective Identification: The Fate of a Concept*. London: Routledge.

Ferro, A. (2006) Clinical Implications of Bion's Thoughts. *International Journal of Psychoanalysis* 87:989–1003.

Ferro, A. and Basile, R. (2009) The Universe of the Field and its Inhabitants. In Ferro, A. and Basile, R. (eds.), *The Analytic Field*. London: Karnac.

Gardner, R. (1983) *Self-reflection*. Boston, MA: Little Brown.

Gerson, S. (2004) The Relational Unconscious. *Psychoanalytic Quarterly* 73(1):63–98.

Green, A. (1986) *On Private Madness*. London: Hogarth.

Heimann, P. (1950) On Counter-Transference. *International Journal of Psychoanalysis* 31:81–84.

Hinz, H. (2012) Projective Identification: The fate the Concept in Germany. In Spillius, E. and O'Shaughnessy, E. (eds.), *Projective Identification: The Fate of a Concept*. London: Routledge.

Jacobs, T.J. (1999) Countertransference Past and Present. *International Journal of Psychoanalysis* 80(3):575–594.

Jacobs, T. (2001) On Unconscious Communications and Covert Enactments: Some Reflections on their Role in the Analytic Situation. *Psychoanalytic Inquiry* 21(1): 4–23.

LaFarge, L. (2007) Commentary on "The Meanings and uses of Countertransference," by Heinrich Racker. *Psychoanalytic Quarterly* 76:795–815.

Ogden, T.H. (1997) Reverie and Interpretation. *Psychoanalytic Quarterly* 66: 567–595.

Pine, F. (2001) Listening and Speaking Psychoanalytically—with What in Mind? *International Journal of Psychoanalysis* 82:901–916.

Pine, F. (2006) The Psychoanalytic Dictionary: A Position Paper on Diversity and its Unifiers. *Journal of the American Psychoanalytic Association* 54:463–491.

Pine, F. (2011) Beyond Pluralism: Psychoanalysis and the Workings of Mind. *Psychoanalytic Quarterly* 80(4):823–856-.

Racker, H. (1953) A Contribution to the Problem of Counter-Transference. *International Journal of Psychoanalysis* 34:313–324.

Racker, H. (1957) The Meanings and Uses of Countertransference. *Psychoanalytic Quarterly* 26:303–357.

Reich, A. (1951) On Counter-Transference. *International Journal of Psychoanalysis* 32:25–31.

Spillius, E. (1992) Clinical Experiences of Projective Identification. In Anderson, R. (ed.), *Clinical Lectures on Klein and Bion*, 59–73. London/New York: Tavistock/Routledge.

Tuch, R. (2015) The Analyst's Way of Being: Recognizing Separable Subjectivities and the Pendulum's Swing. *Psychoanalytic Quarterly* 84:363–388.

Viderman, S. (1974) Interpretation in the Analytical Space. *International Review of Psychoanalysis* 1:467–480.

Waska, R. (2016) The Flexible Function of the Modern Kleinian Psychoanalytic Approach: Interpreting Through the Unbearable Security of Paranoid and Depressive Phantasies. *American Psychoanalytic Association* 76(3):219–223.

6 The External Transferences

In PEP, there are only 7 references to "external transference" and over 42,000 references to "transference",[1] which clearly speaks to how the use of the external transference in analysis has been viewed. Forty years ago, Blum (1983) cogently pointed out that "Extratransference interpretation in psychoanalysis seems to have been relegated to a psychoanalytic limbo in discussions of the theory and practice of psychoanalysis" (p. 587), and it's my impression there has been no change since then. Stone and Halbert (1984) took a strong stand regarding the importance of external transferences. In reflecting on these questions, Stone said that "the patient's responses to the formidable contingencies of life, often revealing affective material not available in the analytic situation, must often be interpreted in the patient's extra-therapeutic life, whether or not clearly related to the transference. Even when a seemingly extra-transferential interpretation is made, it may be, or lead to, an actual transference interpretation by reflexive reference, especially when it involves the patient's intimates. Nonetheless, Stone stated, that there are situations in which transferences themselves may spontaneously occur in the patient's immediate life without evident processing through the analytic situation, and interpretation of these transferences can provide a significant contribution to the psychoanalytic process beyond their immediate therapeutic effects" (p. 138).

Yet as Smith (2003) noted, "It has become generally recognized across many psychoanalytic schools of thought that transference is ubiquitous, in no way limited to the analytic situation" (p. 1022). Further, Joseph (1985) told of how Klein believed that "for many years transference had been understood in terms of direct references to the analyst, and how only later had it been realized that, for example, such things as reports about everyday life, etc. gave a clue to the unconscious anxieties stirred up in the transference situation" (p. 447).[2] Couch (2002) has a different view, saying that "based on a theoretical shift to internal objects and infantile phantasies, new techniques were introduced by the English School that advocated early and constant interpretations of the transference (within the room) from the very start of an analysis" (p. 66, parentheses added).

DOI: 10.4324/9781032658704-8

Since there are so few references to this term in the psychoanalytic literature, with no definition given, the question needs to be asked, "What do I mean by an external transference?" What I'm referring to are the *emotional transferences* an analysand has to the many people he's involved with, in conjunction with the unconscious fantasies enacted with these same people. These include spouses, partners, family members, co-workers, and the myriad other affect-laden, conflictual relationships that come about in living a life. In addition, there are temporary external transferences that might take place with a person in a shop, someone sitting next to the analysand on a plane, a fellow hiker, and so on. Why do I call these relationships outside the analytic setting *transferences*? The transferences in analysis are named so because the analysand transfers his own warded-off unconscious fantasies and aspects of unconscious conflicts on to the analyst, or a warded-off feeling about someone from his past is projected onto the analyst. Is there any doubt that throughout a good part of most analyses, these external relationships are where the patient's *emotions* are *most felt*, and the same mechanisms we see in transferences to the analyst are relived in these relationships? Every possible wish, fantasy, conflict, defense, and so on that dominate patients' views of their analyst exist in relationships outside of the analytic one. These external relationships are where the *patient's affects are, and most intensively felt during long phases in the analysis.* Further, since most analysts would agree that any intervention the analyst makes needs to have an affective valence for the patient if it is to be meaningful, then these external relationships would seem to serve as an ideal place for analytic exploration. Further, I have noticed that many patients are more accepting of interpretations of the external transference than interpretations of the transference onto the analyst until later in the treatment. It is human nature to feel more uncomfortable talking about thoughts and feelings to the person across from you than to someone at a distance. This is especially true with sexual, aggressive, and tender feelings (especially between men).

Freud, throughout most of his writings, believed transference was not just the *most important* but in fact the *only* method by which a genuine psychoanalytic cure could be achieved. Freud believed that the patient seeks to put his passions into action without taking any account of the real situation (p. 108). As Blum (1983) observed, over time, the transference succeeded the dream and became the new "royal road" to the unconscious. However, it hasn't always been noted that late in his career, Freud himself noted some difficulty connected with his formulation of the exclusive role of the analysis of the transference in accounting for therapeutic efficacy (Abend, 2009, p. 872). It is also interesting that from early on he acknowledged that transferences are not unique to psychoanalytic therapy; they arise in all relationships (ibid., p. 874).

The Current Problem with Transference Interpretations

Few psychoanalysts would disagree with the importance of transference interpretations to the success of the treatment. *I would add, however, this is only true if a transference interpretation is made at a time when the analysand can experience the transference as emotionally experienced in the present, while being capable of intellectually understanding it.* It's my sense that if these requirements aren't met transference interpretations are only understood intellectually, and are generally used by patients defensively, if at all.

In general, I find analysts *looking for the transference rather than finding it. We tend to be more eager to bring the transference into the room, rather than finding it in the room.* For instance, when the patient is talking about some interaction outside the consulting room, and the analyst asks, "I wonder if this has to do with you and me", the transference may be forced into the neighborhood rather than allowing it to be there. We seem to believe that unless we are addressing the transference, we aren't doing real analytic work. However, our patients often seem bewildered by many interpretations of the transference, and thus one of the most powerful tools of the analytic method becomes something *imposed and alienating* rather than experienced. We make far too many transference interpretations, too quickly, resulting in an intellectualized appreciation or outright rejection.[3] I have the impression that some analysts, by focusing primarily on the transference, ease the complex task of listening to the analysand's associations. That is, if the analyst has one chord he's listening for, all the other chords making the *symphony of the mind* are screened out, easing the analyst's burden of listening polyphonically.

Green (1974) exposed an important problem with excessive transference interpretations in the following way:

> it is important to realize that an analysis conducted solely through interpretations of the transference often puts the patient under unbearable pressure. The analysis takes on an aspect of persecution even if these interpretations are designed to help the patient understand what is happening within him. The respect for the patient's resistance is one condition of the development of the analytical process. It is sometimes necessary for the patient to project on to the analyst, i.e., to get inside him in order to see what is happening there; but it is also essential that from time to time both look together towards a third object.
>
> (p. 416)

Here is an example where a senior Kleinian analyst (Bott-Spillius, 1994) interprets everything the patient says as a reference to the transference. The analyst notes that the patient responds to these interpretations like a "bewildered child". After briefly wondering if she confronted the patient too brusquely, it's clear she sees it as a problem of the patient rather than a problem with the interpretations. She then goes on to interpret in the same manner. It is also an example of what I've described as the analyst interpreting what may be deeply unconscious, while not paying attention to what may be preconsciously available (in the neighborhood).

> Picking up in the middle of a session the week before the analyst's vacation the patient mentions being pleased to have found a nice cleaning woman. The analyst said, "The good cleaning woman was perhaps a substitute for the bad analyst, who wasn't going to be cleaning her up during the holiday" (p. 1123). The patient then described redecorating her loo (bathroom) and described in detail her plan to buy a mahogany seat.
> The analyst said, "The loo here does not have a mahogany seat. But there is one room here in which there is a lot of mahogany."
> "Oh," she said, "You mean here in this room." She looked carefully around the room. "Yes," she said. "This room is full of mahogany."
> [The analyst then said,] "When you stress that your loo seat is to be made of mahogany, it's as If you are shifting the mahogany from the consulting room into the loo."
> "Oh," she said. (I felt like as if I was spelling things out to an interested but rather bewildered child. Was she really so unaware of what she was saying, I wondered to myself, or had I confronted her too brusquely? It was one of the few occasions up to this time that I was aware of the "obliviousness" that she said other people sometimes complained of."
> "And so," I went on, "You are putting the consulting room into the loo, flushing me and your analysis away. I'm the much-valued cleaner, but when it's the last week of our sessions, I'm flushed away. It's not a case of my leaving you; it's a case of your flushing me away."
>
> (pp. 1123–1124)

This example, where the analyst is seemingly motivated by her theory, every utterance of the patient is perused for its symbolic, unconscious, transference implication. The main problem is that the analyst then interprets to the patient as if these potential symbols of the transference were the same as conscious references to the treating analyst. From my perspective, while the analyst sees the patient as flushing the analyst and analysis down the toilet, I see the analyst as flushing the patient's capacity to convey her story down the toilet. I think many analysts would want to hold in abeyance any thoughts they might have about the patient's statement that she was pleased to find a good cleaning woman until they heard more from the patient.

In the analyst's approach, there seems to be less attention to the readiness of the patient to *hear* and *understand* the analyst's interpretation of the possible symbolic meaning of what she (the patient) may be saying about the treatment. The analyst's ability to read the symbols becomes confused with the patient's ability to understand. This paves the way for the patient to seem like a bewildered child.

It is striking that even after the analyst senses that the patient does not understand, she continues to interpret deeply. The analyst not only pushes these ideas into the room; she also deprives the patient of hosting them. While the analyst interprets the patient's wish to flush her away, the analyst seems to push aside that part of the patient's mind responsible for integrating and synthesizing interpretations.

External Transference Interpretations

Dr. H, a university professor in her late 30s, spoke in her analysis in an assertive manner, much as I imagined she would in lecturing to her university students. She always talked about reality events and didn't have spontaneous associations that could surprise her. Mostly she talked of how others didn't take her into account or appreciate her. This included her children, husband, and colleagues.

Dr. H's parents were trained as engineers, and both had responsible positions in their respective companies. However, it was clear that Dr. H's mother ruled the house, and her father was presented as a schlemiel.[4] It was difficult to get a clear picture of Dr. H's early years, especially who her caretaker was after her mother went back to work, and what age she was when this happened.

In the analysis, I realized Dr. H found it difficult to take in and use my clarifications and interpretations. She might consciously accept what I said, but as she continued speaking, I couldn't find how what I said affected her. It was, as if, what I said was an interruption to what she wanted to talk about. This understanding of what was happening in the sessions only became clear to me after some time. Before this realization, I was most often confused as to how Dr. H had gotten to what she was talking about after I made a clarification or interpretation. At some point, I said, "It's my impression that when I say something that tries to convey my understanding of what you're saying, you accept it, but I don't see that it has any effect upon what you then think." After a brief pause, Dr. H talked of how hurt she was by what I said. After a pause, I told her that I was sorry my impression hurt her feelings but wondered if she could help me understand what she felt hurt by. She explained to me that she believed she was saying what came to mind, like I suggested, and then I told her she was doing it wrong. I said I could see how that could be confusing but reminded her that one way I tried to understand her was to see what she did with her thoughts.

(As the reader can see there are two ways I respond to Dr. H that consider her narcissistic vulnerability. In my first reaction to her feeling hurt, I thought it was important to apologize, not for what I said, but that she felt my comment hurt her. Secondly, I thought it important to confirm her idea that it could seem like I was giving her confusing messages. My further explanation was my attempt to bring in the reality of the analytic task before us as a way of seeing if she could stand back and look at her reaction in a different way. However, she remained feeling hurt. I understand, now, that this interpretation of an enacted transference in language action was premature, and had elements of a countertransference enactment on my part. I was aware of Dr. H's narcissistic vulnerability to comments from anyone that she wasn't doing something exactly right. In retrospect, I can see how my frustration over how I often felt confused in listening to her was not well contained. Further evidence of my countertransference reaction was that I'd already written about how the analysand's use of language action is unconscious, and I don't believe what's unconscious can be approached directly.

After the above incident, I avoided making clarifications or interpretations based upon what I thought was happening in the here and now of the session. At a certain point I thought of Dr. H's relationship with her husband as an example of another man whom she had difficulty listening to or investing in. For many years, if her husband was mentioned at all, she would complain bitterly about his meanness and lack of appreciation for her. An incident at his work made it clear he was also greatly admired and liked by other faculty and his students. It was then I could wonder with Dr. H about her one-sided view of her husband. It's an example of how external events can help explain an internal transference. This eventually led to her seemingly appreciating her husband more, and then he disappeared from view. What I mean by this is that Dr. H would describe vacations with her children or family outings, with no mention of her husband. At one point, when Dr. H was describing a family trip, she only talked about her interactions with her children. I wondered if her husband was on this trip. She answered in the affirmative, and I said I asked because on most of the trips she talks about, it's been my impression that her husband isn't mentioned. She replied defensively that she thought it was clear because she described them as family trips. I said I could see that, but what I was describing was that she never mentioned any interaction with her husband on these trips.

Over time she became more open to my comments about her relationship with her husband. What seemed to help most was when she continually complained about her husband, I would empathize with her feelings, but I also reminded her of what she had told me previously, of how many people admired and valued her husband, and how she never seemed to see this side of him. This seemed to cause Dr. H to allow me some space to start to examine her relationship with her husband. I could help her see the various ways she needed to have her husband mirror her, and how angry she became when this didn't happen. I told her I thought this was understandable as she seemed to miss this experience in her growing up.[5] As she began to understand and accept her anger, there was a change in how she consciously experienced me. For the first time, she was able to express how she appreciated what I was helping her understand, and also expressed disappointment that we weren't meeting when there was a holiday. Her behavior in the sessions started to change also. For the first time she was able to laugh at herself for the way she was, told jokes, and reported dreams, where erotic wishes towards me could be talked about. I believed at this point she'd be more able to tolerate my clarifying that part of her that could still be dismissive of me. In one session when she talked about how angry she was with her son for his post-modern views, I said that I could understand that she disagreed with him, but I wondered if we could think about why it made her angry. Her thoughts went to an aunt she stayed with one summer, and how critical she felt she was. This aunt was a stickler for language and would correct Dr. H's grammar at times. She said she felt so "embarrassed". She felt this aunt was very critical of her the whole summer. I then said to Dr. H that I could appreciate she might not appreciate her aunt's comments but wondered about this feeling of embarrassment. At a certain point she came back to my question and said, in passing, that it was a dumb question since, of course she felt embarrassed. I wondered if she could see the possibility that she was critical and dismissive of my question. She briefly acknowledged this and brought up how many scholars wrote about Philip Roth's conflicted feelings about women. She then mentioned how one prominent critic dismissed these speculations as explanatory, since many men have conflicted feelings about women, but not everyone becomes a Philip Roth. Then I said, "So your thoughts go to a prominent thinker who dismissed psychological explanation." Dr. H's response was that she could see what I might make of this, but she wasn't aware of feeling dismissive. I then said, "It seems possible you're dismissive of my saying you were being dismissive, using an explanation that dismisses the very basis of our work, which is that there are forces you aren't conscious of sometimes that may drive your thoughts and feelings."[6] She became more contemplative after this and felt she could now hear what I was saying. There was then a brief pause, and Dr. H then launched into a description of an issue that was being considered at her university, and her views about it. I couldn't see anything in what she was saying that was related to the issue of her dismissiveness, and I thought this was the point; that is, again she was dismissing what I had brought up with her. I also considered that her thoughts were a defense against a painful awareness. As the end of the session was imminent, I decided to not say anything at this point.

On the following day, Dr. H didn't mention anything about the issue of dismissiveness, or the day after. At some point I mentioned that the issue of being dismissive seemed to have disappeared from her mind. After a brief pause, she said that, in fact, later in the day of the session we talked about it, she was trying to remember what the session was about but drew a blank. She then put it out of her mind. Dr. H went on to say that she guessed one could say she dismissed what we had talked about. I could hear the disowning of her statement as she said it, that is, when she phrased her thought as "she *guessed one* could say…". Her use of the term "one" leaves it vague as to who this person is, while presenting this as a "guess" makes it less definitive that she believes this idea that she was being dismissive. I then wondered with her if she could hear the vagueness in who owned this guess. She then said, "I guess I can" and laughed with a recognition that she used this "disowning" word. She wondered why she was being so defensive as she could see how dismissive she could be. It was the end of the session and I said, "that is an important question".

In this vignette, we can see how by first focusing on the external transference leads to an understanding of Dr. H's internal transference. However, I want to reiterate that for a certain amount of time, patients are more comfortable with interpretations based on the external transference. I believe it is only later in an analysis that we can make *usable* interpretations of the internal transference.

Notes

1   A perusal of these articles indicates they are describing transferences onto the analyst.
2   Strachey (1934) captured what, according to Joseph, must have been Klein's earlier views, when he stated, "we now turn back and consider for a little the picture I have given of a mutative interpretation with its various characteristics, we shall notice that my description appears to exclude every kind of interpretation except those of a single class—the class, namely, of *transference* interpretations. Is it to be understood that no extra-transference interpretation can set in motion the chain of events which I have suggested as being the essence of psycho-analytical therapy?" (p. 154).

3   I am reminded of the old joke where an author is talking to another guest at a social gathering. After a while, the author apologizes for going on about himself and suggests that he'd like to hear about the other person and asks, "So what did you think of my most recent book?"
4   Yiddish for an inept person.
5   In general, I find it helpful for patients to see their thoughts, feelings, and actions as, in part, a normal response to abnormal conditions.
6   With our actions, we hope to bring back into operation a working ego.

References

Abend, S. M. (2009) Freud, Transference, and Therapeutic Action. *Psychoanalytic Quarterly* 78:871–892.

Blum, H. (1983) The Position and Value of Extra-transference Interpretation. *Journal of the American Psychoanalytic Association* 31:587–617.

Bott-Spillius, E. (1994) On Formulating Clinical fact to the Patient. *International Journal of Psychoanalysis* 75: 1121–1132.

Couch, A. S. (2002) Extra-Transference Interpretation: A Defense of Classical Technique. *Psychoanalytic Study of the Child* 57:63–92.

Green, A. (1974) Surface Analysis, Deep Analysis (The Role of the Preconscious in Psychoanalytical Technique). *International Review of Psychoanalysis* 1:415–423.

Joseph, B. (1985) Transference: The Total Situation. *International Journal of Psychoanalysis.* 66:447–454.

Smith, H.F. (2003) Analysis of Transference: A North American perspective. *International Journal of Psychoanalysis* 84:1017–1041.

Stone, L. and Halpert, E. (1984) The Value of Extratransference Interpretation. *Journal of the American Psychoanalytic Association* 32:137–146.

Strachey, J. (1934) The Nature of the Therapeutic Action of Psycho-Analysis. *International Journal of Psychoanalysis* 15:127–159.

7 Self-Criticism as an Unconscious Lifeline

There is a type of patient one sees in psychoanalysis where *criticism surrounds them like a cloud*. There have been numerous dynamic explanations for this, but what I hope to show in this chapter is that the patients I'm describing *are driven by a different*, but not unrelated dynamic to what has been described before. Patients who feel the need for criticism as a *lifeline* seem to have experienced a mother who is viewed as the more *powerful* parent, and is idealized as intelligent, competent, and/or beautiful and charming. The child's basic physical needs are provided for. However, most striking is that the mother is experienced *primarily as emotionally absent, and that her main affective connection with the child came via being critical.* A child's tendency towards egocentric thinking leads him to wonder what's he's done wrong that leads the mother to be so distant and leads to a life-long unconscious identification as someone who is "difficult", a "freak", or in more extreme cases, "hated". What emerges over time in these patients' transferences is the way they silently take the analyst's observations as criticism, and if they can't help but experience the analyst as helpful, they "know" the analyst really thinks of them more critically. While support of their healthy narcissism is necessary, it does not help the patient in the long run as it threatens their inner connection to the one and only lively primary object, that is, the critical mother.

A good example can be seen at the beginning of a session with a patient who has enough awareness, at this point, to observe the way he is drawn to self-criticism, and anticipating criticism from others.

Patient: Did you give me a bill last time? I couldn't remember. I searched all around the house but couldn't find it. I thought you must have given it to me, and I felt like a real fuck-up. Then I realized I could bring my checkbook and pay you, but then I forgot my pen.

(Here one can see the degree of self-criticism that is already attached to the analyst and the session. As this ever-present self-criticism is something we've been talking about, I start to feel critical towards Mr. A for not relating what he just described to this, then realize he is inviting me to think critically about him.)

FB: So, you come in already connected with me via self-criticism.

DOI: 10.4324/9781032658704-9

Patient: I can see how critical of myself I am, *but sometimes I think I'm not critical enough.*

FB: So, you're critical of yourself for not being critical enough.

Patient: Funny, or maybe not so funny, as soon as you started talking, I had an image of my mother's face as she was criticizing me for still another thing I hadn't done the way she would have liked me to do it.

Of course, patients who are self-critical and anticipating criticism have been known about for some time in psychoanalysis. The basis for what I'll be outlining can, and I think needs to be differentiated from those patients wracked by guilt, suffering from melancholia, or who rely primarily on projection as a defense. However, there are shades of each as part of the symptom picture. Thus, while the symptoms in the patients I'll describe are similar to other forms of pathology where criticism is prominent, I hope to show that the underlying causes are different. The patient's identification with the mother's critical view (as the difficult or hated one), and who anticipates criticism from others, keeps the mother present and serves as a form of *ground zero for the patient's stable connection to life.* When not experiencing criticism, these patients experience the fear of a *terrifying void.* This is what makes the identifications so difficult to give up. Its identification as a *lifeline* is central to the outcome of the treatment.

The Patient Picture

In general, these patients I'll be describing first appear as functioning neurotics. Like others in this category, they seem to do well enough professionally and have stable relationships (characterized by criticism), but get little pleasure in their accomplishments, whether professionally or interpersonally. While this picture characterizes many patients we see in our practices, the specifics are different for these patients. For example, Mr. A came to treatment after an anxiety attack when he won a prestigious award in his field. Over time, it emerged that at *that* moment he could no longer see himself primarily as an "annoying little kid" and *had frightening images of being alone on an isolated island in the middle of a vast ocean. Something similar to this dread of being totally cut off from human contact is what leads to the patient's need to desperately cling to self-criticism or unconsciously induce criticism from others.* It is a way to hold on to the primary object. It is different from melancholia, where self-criticism is based on criticism of an object turned inward. With the patients I'm describing, self-criticism is based on a primary object's criticism, plus the child's fantasies of why the primary object is so cold toward them.

What emerges over time in these patients' transferences is the way they silently take the analyst's observations as criticism, and if they can't help but experience the analyst as helpful, they "know" the analyst really thinks of them more critically. While support of their healthy narcissism is necessary, it does not help the patient in the long run as it threatens their inner connection to the one and only lively primary object, that is, the critical mother.

In my countertransference reaction to these patients, what might ordinarily seem like a defensive reaction or small rebellion against the frame has left me feeling denigrated and led me to make observations with a critical tone. In addition to unconsciously inviting criticism, it is an identification with the critical mother. Most striking, *these patients don't seem particularly upset when I enact a countertransference reaction by expressing something with a critical tone, and even welcome it*. When I'm able to step back and say something like, "It seemed to me that there was a certain sarcasm in what I just said", the patient acknowledges hearing it but dismisses the idea that it was meant critically (i.e., a lifeline has been established and can't be broken). From another perspective, these patients may act in ways that bring about criticism. For example, one patient's body odor was so bad I had to use an air cleaner during sessions. These patients also have difficulty experiencing love or praise, as it threatens their lifeline. When the analyst points to a discrepancy between the patient's perception of her world as critical (e.g., colleagues at work) and what seems like her colleagues' support and praise, the observation is rushed past in a torrent of words that leaves the analyst befuddled as to how we got to this point, and thus he becomes *self-critical for his inability* to understand his patient.

What emerges over time is that the patient comes to realize he becomes anxious and is silently dismissing anything the analyst might say that appears to have even *the slightest positive element*. The patient's anxiety might be seen in a mental startle reaction that leaves the patient briefly silent before associating to some way he acted badly or was reacted to badly.

While initially the patient presents a picture of his mother as "good enough", over time the patient reports comments that mother has made to the patient that seem very critical and demeaning. The patient seems to have no reaction to these comments and remains close to his mother. When the analyst first observes that some people might take such remarks as critical, the patient sloughs it off with comments like, "She means well", or "She was saying it for my own good". Over time it becomes clear that there is severe anxiety associated with even observing, let alone questioning, the patient's connection with his critical mother.

It is not uncommon for the analyst to believe that the patient unconsciously married someone just like his or her mother or worse, and wonder why he/she stays in the relationship. It is only after understanding the patient's need for self-criticism that one begins to sense there are ways the patient brings about criticism and is critical and dismissive of the spouse. Early attempts to help the patient search for the cause of his self-criticism will most often lead to the intensification of the patient's self-criticism as his "badness" has been discovered.

A Writer's Nightmare

Elizabeth Tallent, a gifted short-story writer, didn't publish anything for 20 years because of withering self-criticism. In her attempt to open a window into her long silence, she describes "my long confinement in closed-circuit viciousness designating every attempt *error fuckup hideous miscarriage*" (Tallent, 2020, p. 9). Her background is like I've described with my patients. Her mother tells her at age nineteen that she didn't want her, and that the nurses kept trying to have her mother hold and feed her, which the mother refused. Tallent's perspective of how her mother told the story gives a sense of their relationship over the years. "What she was telling me appeared to strike her as a strange story involving only herself, unlikely to have any effect on me" (ibid., p. 30). The mother's explanation was that she didn't look like the baby on the Gerber's baby food jar, which she hadn't realized was a six-month-old baby. Throughout the mother's telling of the story, Tallent constantly experiences her own loathsomeness. She describes how "often my sense was whatever I became self-conscious about, she (her mother) had for some time been critically aware of" (ibid., p. 29, parenthesis added).

As with the patients I've described, Tallent's mother was not only critical. She was attractive, lively in company, and loved by her husband for her wittiness and reserve. He needed her approval. However, she was "vulnerable to becoming entranced by hostility, once she had started in on someone or other's slighting behavior, she could be consumed by wrongs, her exaggerated woundedness often made it hard to figure out the truth of what you were hearing. In a double dose of misfortune, Tallent's father was also very critical. Tallent achingly describes looking for affirmation that never comes, and like many children, blames herself. "The truth is I was sickened by myself for being a child they wanted not to know about. I repudiated myself because I could find no way to matter" (p. 68), and later on, "I was imbued with wrongness, irretrievably wrong, a wrong self, and that could not be changed, and it could not be borne" (p. 68).

In short, the emotionally absent mother who was present for Tallent only when she was delivering withering criticism was typical for my patients. Further, echoing my patients' experience, the anticipation of *loss* looms as the greatest fear in relinquishing self-criticism. Thus, Tallent notes in passing a study where the authors suggest that what keeps this maladaptive self-criticism going is that without it, "It would result in some other form of substantial loss, such as losing or disrupting an important relational connection" (ibid., p. 10).

Relevant Historical Antecedents

In this section, I present contributions from the literature that are descriptively similar to what I've described but have a different dynamic picture.

All writing on this topic began with Freud's (1917) paper on "Mourning and Melancholia", although Strachey (1957) notes in his introduction to the paper that in an 1897 letter to Fliess, Freud remarkably already laid out the dynamics he was to elaborate some years later.

Freud's paper is so well known I will not dwell on it except to remind us of some of his key observations.

> The distinguishing mental features of melancholia are a profoundly painful dejection … inhibition of all activity, and a lowering of the self-regarding feelings to a degree *that finds utterance in self-reproaches and self-revilings and culminates in a delusional expectation of punishment.* This picture becomes a little more intelligible when we consider that, with one exception, the same traits are met with in mourning. *The disturbance of self-regard is absent in mourning;* but otherwise, the features are the same.
>
> (p. 244, italics added.)

Freud then explains that the melancholic's intense self-criticisms

> are hardly at all applicable to the patient himself, but that with insignificant modifications they do fit someone else, *someone whom the patient loves or has loved or should love.* Every time one examines the facts this conjecture is confirmed. So, we find the key to the clinical picture: we perceive that the self-reproaches are reproaches against a loved object which have been shifted away from it on to the patient's own ego.
>
> (p. 248, italics added)

Freud explains what happens based upon a split in the ego, where one part sets itself against the other, and critically judges it. Freud expounds on this by offering that "an attachment of the libido to a particular person, had at one time existed; then, owing to a real slight or disappointment coming from this loved person, the object-relationship was shattered" (ibid., p. 249). He continues his explanation based upon what happens to the withdrawn libido after such a disappointment. That is, the libido was not then attached to another object, but withdrawn into the ego, leading to an identification of the ego with the abandoned object. In one of his most memorable statements, he states that thus the "shadow of the object fell upon the ego" (ibid., p. 248), and the latter could henceforth be judged by a special agency, as though it were an object, the forsaken object.

> In this way an object-loss was transformed into an ego-loss and the conflict between the ego and the loved person into a cleavage between the critical activity of the ego and the ego as altered by identification.
>
> (ibid., p. 249)

Freud sees intense ambivalence toward the love object as a crucial element in the formation of melancholia.

In the patients I'm discussing, the symptom picture is not so severe as in melancholia. Their self-criticism is more subtle, and *not* mainly directed toward the ambivalently held object, while a *critical attitude toward others seems primarily designed to invite criticism,* which the analyst will find ample evidence of in his countertransference. Depression is a low-level affect in the background of their lives, but they are generally active people, sometimes as a defense.

Fairbairn (1952) introduced the term "moral defense" for the patient who takes on the feeling of badness, which appears to originally reside in his objects. By doing this, the patient attempts to purge the badness in his objects and feels a sense of security in a world of good objects.

> The child would rather be bad himself than have bad objects. ... In becoming bad he is really taking upon himself the burden of badness which appears to reside in his objects. By this means he seeks to purge them of their badness; and, in proportion as he succeeds in doing so, he is rewarded by that sense of security which an environment of good objects so characteristically confers.
>
> (Fairbairn, 1952, p. 64)

In the patients I'm describing, it is a frightening feeling of *aloneness* that they fear, not the loss of a sense of security if the patient recognizes the world is populated by bad objects.

In an important but neglected article, Valenstein (1973) wrote about patients *who were attached to pain.* While he emphasized that these patients were mostly attached to psychical pain, he suggested this could also be physical pain. He saw the attachment to pain as stemming from *object ties within the first year of life*, signifying an original attachment to painfully experienced objects that are also *inconsistent in* their connection to the infant. He saw this very early history as an essential element in the negative therapeutic reaction. Valenstein gives an example where

> a colicky infant may be inclined toward "pain" and *Unlust* in the same way as an infant in whom pain was induced from the outside. If a mother of a discomforted and restless infant then adds to the mother–child misfit, either because of her own incompetency or because of reciprocal difficulties, an increasing structurization of a set toward pain as the predominant affect connoting self and object is likely to emerge in the child.
>
> (ibid., p. 373)

He believes that for these patients, *getting better is dreaded*. A patient of Valenstein's describes the fear of being without pain in a beautiful but terrifying manner.

> "I don't know how to do without it—this constant pain. Without it I would have nothing, and if I gave it up it would be like being different and like falling off a chair into space and being terrifyingly alone".
>
> (p. 388)

This danger in recovery, based upon feeling "terrifyingly alone", is characteristic of the patients I'm describing. An almost intractable negative therapeutic reaction in the patient's Valenstein describes has only been a small part of my patients' reactions and can be worked through once *the way* the patient is experiencing the analyst can be better articulated in the transference. Further, I have not seen the attachment to self-criticism in the patients I'll describe as stemming primarily from the first year of life. In fact, these patients generally function well in their profession, which is most often correlated with a relatively healthy part of their ego associated with the "good-enough" *early* mother.

Shengold (1989) noted something similar to what I've seen in his "soul murder" patients, who "survived their childhood with considerable intactness" (p. 310), and even showed a great many strengths. In Shengold's (1978a, 1978b, 1989) explication of the conditions for "soul murder", he describes a dynamic during childhood that is similar to what I've outlined with my patients. Shengold describes a situation where a parent enacts "a regimen of cruelty and seduction (overstimulation) with indifference and neglect (deprivation) that provides the environmental matrix for soul murder" (1978a, p. 419). He

added that the child must deal with what has happened by not knowing, not acknowledging, not remembering (1978b). He focused on
these patients' distrust of others based on projections of anger based
on the aggressive drives and fears of losing control, but also *"experienced* reality" (Shengold, 1978b, p. 312). Shengold sees rage as an
import part of the picture. He describes how massive defenses against
all deep feelings and meaningful relationships are aroused because of
the danger of the rage breaking through and turning inward toward
great guilt and a need to be punished.

While overstimulation, as described by Shengold, has been part of
the picture in some patients, it is not a consistent factor. What I do
find is when the primary object isn't emotionally available, she can
appear lively and attractive, especially with an appreciative audience,
suggesting the narcissistic pathology underlying her behavior. While
projected anger is part of the picture with my patients, it isn't based
on an aggressive drive, and it isn't defended against because of fear
of it breaking through, but rather because of the fear of losing the
lifeline.

Anton Kris has written extensively on patients where self-criticism
is a central factor in their pathology, but to my reading most succinctly captured this in a 1990 publication. He convincingly correlates
unconscious self-criticism with narcissistic pathology and delineates
how the narcissist's excessive demands for narcissistic gratification can
be based upon unconscious self-criticism of these same demands that
makes any need suspect. Thus, what these patients desire they cannot
get based on guilt over these same wishes. This leads to an unending
feeling of deprivation which increases the need for satisfaction. This
self-criticism is always externalized onto the analyst. He reviews how
narcissism and self-criticism were reinforced by earlier *analytic* attitudes and approvingly notes how Kohut's approach of an "affirmative
attitude" characterized by acceptance, acknowledgment, or affirmation by recognition always replaces rejection or criticism. In fact, Kris
believes an "affirmative attitude, far from being a substitute for resistance analysis, is the *sine qua non* when punitive self-critical attitudes
run high" (Kris, 1990, p. 621).

The patients I'm describing are also unable to gratify wishes, and
narcissistic elements are present *to various degrees*. However, they are
not the clamoring narcissists one sees when narcissistic deprivation is
primary. Instead, these patients deny themselves many things which
might give them pleasure in life but feel virtuous about this rather than
deprived.

One way to differentiate the patients I'm describing from those
described in the Kleinian *paranoid-schizoid* position is that the paranoid-schizoid patients are viewed as within the range of borderline
character disorders (Hinshelwood, 1991). Their readiness to feel
attacked is the result of projection, with a weakened ego, that makes

them more volatile. In the one instance I could find where Klein (1958) specifically described self-criticism, she linked it with binding the death instinct which influences "the aspects of the good objects contained in the superego, with the result that the action of the superego ranges from restraint of hate and destructive impulses, protection of the good object and self-criticism, to threats, inhibitory complaints and persecution." One can see here that she was describing the healthier aspects of self-criticism. In the *depressive position,* Klein, much like Freud, saw ambivalence toward an internal object, experienced as within the self, creating "a crisis over one's sense of self—in particular there ensues a self-condemnation and self-hatred" (Hinshelwood and Fortuna, 2018, p. 65). Descriptively, this is a more extreme version of what my patients experience. Further, it is based on the patient desperately holding on to the primary object's highly cathected negative view of him/her that is central to the self-criticism.

Andre Green's (2001) descriptions of the *moral masochist and moral narcissist* come closest to the patients I'm describing. They have elements of each. As he describes it, "The true moral narcissist always volunteers himself whenever he sees a chance to renounce satisfaction" (ibid., p. 13), while the moral masochist's inner world is filled with fantasies of being beaten (psychically and physically) and humiliated. The moral narcissist demands love, and sees the path for receiving it, via the *others' recognition of their denunciation of pleasure.* The moral masochist experiences pain and humiliation constantly, and unconsciously seeks it out. While Green sees it as useful to separate these two -character traits, he doesn't see them as entirely separate. This fits with the patients I'm describing.

Clinical Example

This is the full vignette of my work with the patient described at the beginning of this chapter. As a reminder, the patient came into the session connected to me via self-criticism over what he thought he didn't do (i.e., pay the bill), and generally he felt he wasn't self-critical enough. In my reciprocal countertransference, I began to feel critical of him. As I was talking, an image came to his mind of a particular look on his mother's face when she criticized him. The session continues.

Mr. A: I've been incessantly playing this on-line chess game. I both really enjoy it but feel guilty whenever I play it. Like yesterday I played for an hour before starting work, and then criticized myself for doing it when I have so much to do. It doesn't help that Helen (his wife) also criticizes me for playing chess last night instead of reading in the living room with her.

> *(I found myself thinking that for many years he convincingly portrayed his wife as very critical, but now I can see he may also act in ways that lead to her criticism.)*

Mr. A: I watched a documentary over the holiday on eating a low-protein diet and tried to eat that way for the next week. I really started to feel physically strange. He then started to struggle to explain how he felt, and then told me how he felt he had more energy, felt more virile, went back to the gym, and so on So, it became clear the strange feeling he had was feeling *good*. He then started to question his good feeling as having anything to do with his diet and suggested it was probably a halo effect.

FB: I think it's important that what you label as strange was feeling good, and then were drawn to criticize yourself for thinking this "good" diet had anything to do with what you did.

Mr. A: Then recounted an incident that happened when he was about seven. At a gathering of neighbors, he and his brother were in the corner of a room telling "bathroom" jokes. His mother heard them and started criticizing him in particular and then launched into a number of other grievances she had toward him before she sent him home. His brother wasn't admonished. He was angry with her at first, but then wondered if maybe he unconsciously knew his mother might hear him, and how she disapproved of these jokes.

> *(This seemed like it could be a potential insight, but also a form of self-criticism.)*

The scene of his mother being critical of him or absent had played out through his life. During his early years, his mother was beginning her acting career, and he was cared for by a series of nannies. Most of his interactions with his mother were experienced by him as her pointing out that he was falling short of her expectations. At an earlier time in treatment, I had the feeling that for whatever reason, his mother saw him as a "bad seed". Neither his older brother nor younger brother came in for such criticism. He poignantly remembered trying to figure out how they were behaving and mimicked it in the hopes he could avoid his mother's criticism, but to no avail.

Analyzing Criticism as a Lifeline

How do we begin the analysis of a symptom that is associated with the *terror* of giving up a lifeline? It is the same question we face in analyzing any symptom or character defense, although the frightening feelings vary. Further, how do we differentiate criticism as a lifeline from other forms of self-criticism? I have found that the answer to both questions begin with the under-utilized method of *clarification* in the here and now of the session. Clarification depicts *how* self-criticism takes place, not *why*, thus beginning the process of containment by building representations. By building a *container* via words *we help the patient face the terrifying process of losing a lifeline.* In this way we give the patient a better opportunity to explore the *why* of self-criticism by slowly muting the feeling of terror. As it is more difficult for patients to see how they might invite criticism from others (especially in the transference/countertransference), we start out by helping the patient see how relentlessly self-critical she is. As the patient is likely to take this as a criticism, we need to be alert to the signs of how this occurs. It is only over repeated clarifications that a container is built. It can be helpful if we use analyst-centered clarifications that can aid in minimizing the sting of a clarification that the patient will take as a criticism. It is a variation on Steiner's (1994) analyst-centered interpretations, where the clarification begins with something like "I noticed, or I have the sense that" rather than "You are". For example, we might begin a clarification with "*I* have the impression when someone is critical you seem to accept it" rather than saying, "You readily accept criticism". We hope, that over time, the patient will be able to observe her tendency to self-criticism herself, thus beginning the process of further analysis. At a later point in the analysis, when the ties to self-criticism are not so strong, we can more directly clarify it. Eventually we need the patient's association to help us differentiate the dynamic and genetic understanding of criticism as either a lifeline or some other etiology. Clarification is, of course, only the beginning in analyzing the unconscious dynamics at the basis of self-criticism.

References

Fairbairn, W.R.D. (1952) *Psychoanalytic Studies of the Personality.* London: Tavistock.

Freud, S. (1917) Mourning and Melancholia. *S.E.*: 237–258.

Green, A. (1975) The Analyst's Symbolization and Absence in the Analytic Setting. *Int. J. Psychoanal.*, 56:1–22.

Green, A. (2001) Moral Narcissism. In Green, A. (ed.), *Life Narcissism and Death Narcissism.* London: Free Association Books.

Hinshelwood, R.D. (1991) Review of Psychic Equilibrium and Psychic change by Betty Joseph. *Free Associations*, 2(2):295–310.

Hinshelwood, R.D. and Fortuna, T. (2018) *Melanie Klein the Basics.* London: Routledge.

Klein, M. (1958) On the Development of Mental Functioning. *Int. J. Psycho-Anal.*, 39:84–90.

Kris, A.O. (1990) Helping Patients by Analyzing Self-Criticism. *J. Amer. Psychoanal. Assn.*, 38:605–636.

Shengold, L. (1978a) Assault on a Child's Individuality: A Kind of Soul Murder. *Psychoanal. Q.*, 47:419–424.

Shengold, L. (1978b) Kaspar Hauser and Soul Murder: A Study of Deprivation. *Int. Rev. Psycho-Anal.*, 5:457–476.
Shengold, L. (1989) *Soul Murder*. New York: Ballentine Books.
Steiner, J. (1994) Patient-centered and Analyst-centered Interpretations. *Psychoanal. Inq.*, 14:406–422.
Strachey, J. (1957) Introduction to "Mourning and Melancholia" (1917). *S.E.*: 239.
Tallent, E. (2020) *Scratched*. New York: Harper Collins.
Valenstein, A.F. (1973) On Attachment to Painful Feelings and the Negative Therapeutic Reaction. *Psychoanal. St. Child*, 28:365–392.

8 Silence on Silence

At times, a gifted novelist can capture in a few sentences what those of us writing for a professional audience need multiple pages to explain. Regarding silence, Nicole Kraus (2006), in her beautiful novel *The History of Love,* wrote the following:

> Only after they charged him with the crime of silence did Babel discover how many kinds of silence existed. When he heard music, he no longer listened to the notes, but the silences in between ... When people spoke to him, he heard less and less of what they were saying, and more and more of what they were not.

Silence in the analytic hour is akin to the 180 words Eskimos have for snow; that is, there are a multitude of variations. There is silence as a sign of anxiety, fear, anger, or over-excitement. Silence can be a dream, a reverie, or sleep. It can be a fear of a thought or thinking. It can be a time of reflection, or a moment when the patient retreats from the clamoring in her head. The list goes on. *What I will focus on in this chapter is silence as a rupture in the patient's narrative.* This can occur in various forms. For example, when a patient is talking and suddenly falls silent in the middle of her narrative; when the patient is silent after an analyst's intervention; and when the patient begins a session with a lengthy silence. What characterizes these moments, and others like them, is that the patient's mind has suddenly gone blank, or that she's no longer verbalizing what is on her mind. The analyst's puzzlement in his own mind at these moments (e.g., "What just happened?") is different than when there is a brief pause, or a moment when the patient may be reflecting.

It is my impression from listening to and reading hundreds of case presentations that there are two main ways silences are dealt with. The first is that the silence is treated as an *epiphenomenon,* that is, a secondary event to whatever else may be occurring at the moment in the analytic hour. However, reflection will lead us to understand that this is unlikely to be a secondary event. When a patient suddenly stops her narrative and falls silent, or responds to the analyst's interpretation

DOI: 10.4324/9781032658704-10

with silence, *it would seem evident something has just happened in the patient's mind.*

The second way we often deal with silence is to ask a question about what the patient *isn't talking about.* A not uncommon question in response to silence is, "What are you thinking?" This focuses on the hidden content, and *not the hiddenness itself.* Further, if it were just an issue of asking the right question, why wouldn't the patient just be saying whatever was stopped? It is the hesitation, the reluctance to keep talking, that is the most important issue. With such a question, we bypass the opportunity to help the patient see *that something just happened* in her mind that led her to feel the need to stop.

A not atypical scenario reported by a colleague went like this. In the middle of a session, a patient says, "I'm frustrated", followed by a brief silence, after which the analyst asks, "Can you tell me more about the frustration?" which the patient might do. However, how do we know the silence isn't the most important part of the moment? Does the patient wish to frustrate us as well? Is the patient blaming us for his frustration, or expecting us to do something? Is the patient attempting to suppress the feeling? Is he attempting to stay with the feeling, recognizing the wish to undo it? Is he in a reverie in association with this feeling? Is the silence, dark, demanding, brooding, or blank? There can be so much in the patient saying, "I'm frustrated", and then falling silent. By asking the patient to tell us more about the *frustration,* we bypass the silence that might be the most important part of the narrative. Further, by *rushing in* with a question we may convey our own difficulty in tolerating silence. Asking the patient to tell us more bypasses what the patient spontaneously does in reaction to this feeling of frustration (i.e., silence) which is the most meaningful to the understanding of the patient. Further, we also convey our own comfort with uncomfortable feelings if we can sit in silence waiting for the patient to struggle with what is best for him to do at this moment.

Questions about silence are sometimes presented *as a way of filling in the gaps* in the patient's narrative, but often seem to become a form of interrogation (see Levenson, 1988). From my perspective, *gaps are what is happening in the analysis, not something to be filled in.* As I understand it, *gaps are the openings that leave room for something yet unknown to emerge,* and thus are best understood via an analytic process.

If we believe that one central component of what is curative in psychoanalysis is to help the patient find, or re-find, her mind, ignoring what appears to be a disruptive silence as a psychological event is to bypass a potentially significant transference enactment that has just occurred before us. In general, analysis works best if we consider everything that happens in an analysis as a dream.

An Example from Prague

At an IPA meeting, de Cortiñas (2013, pgs. 537–538) presented a beautiful piece of analytic work from a Bionian perspective with a patient whom she understood as having symbolic failures related to the obstruction of development of phantasies, dreams, dream thoughts, and so on. I present this material not to supervise, but to give an example of how a gifted analysis works with silence in what I see as a typical fashion, and to present an alternative approach that emphasizes the significance of silence as a rupture in the clinical moment. The analyst's experience of the patient (Ana) was that "nothing she did or said seemed to resonate emotionally in me ... She did not laugh, never smiled, nor did she cry or get angry. Everything in our analytic relationship sounded hollow and seemed empty" (p. 536).

My comments on the session will be in italics.

Ana: After yesterday's session, it seems that I don't take care of myself, and what happens to me is because I don't take care.
(Silence)
Analyst: What do you mean by that?

Ana's opening remarks seem to be a result of the analytic work. There is an I that is taking responsibility for her symptoms. She is not blaming others or life but sees herself as the cause of her difficulties. This is a place we hope patients reach. With such a progressive step, there is often anxiety, and I would wonder if this was the cause of her silence. Analysands often wonder, "How will the analyst react to such a step?" After a sufficient period of time elapsed, I might respond in the following manner: "After appreciating how you don't take care of yourself you fall silent, as if something interfered with your going further." Notice I'm not suggesting what the interference might be but am leaving it for the patient to tell me via their associations, or lack thereof, what may come to mind. It is an invitation to reflect rather than asking for an answer. I would call this an unsaturated clarification, *borrowing Ferro's (2002) felicitous phrase, as it isn't directed toward any particular content, dynamic, or part of the mind. Unsaturated clarifications can be characterized as basically saying, "I noticed something. Can you notice it too?" It is an attempt to bring new connections to the patient's mind, without suggesting any direction the patient should take. It may lead to playful musing, diversionary obfuscation, or multiple other responses.*

With the analyst asking, "What did you mean by that?" she directs Ana's attention to the "not taking care of herself" content, while the reason for her falling silent after noticing this is bypassed. Let's see what happens.

Ana: Yesterday I phoned the gynecologist, and I didn't find him, and I have everything swollen. I almost couldn't button my trousers. And I have eczema and my spine. *These are problems of my head.* (italics added)

Ana's response is to someone not *being there for her. It is an association to the analyst's comments, suggesting Ana felt the analyst's response was not helpful. However, she tries again to let the analyst know she has understood her problems are in* her *head.*

Analyst: Your body seems to have problems that your head doesn't understand, unknown, weird, problems: a pregnancy, delivering a baby. Problems that are different from those you know and that you were looking for in Cañada, when you stopped taking the pills.

It seems the analyst is negating the patient's accomplishment. Ana is saying, "I understand these physical symptoms are from my own mind", while the analyst is saying, "Your head doesn't understand these bodily problems".

Ana: (She laughs in a rather childish way. Is she laughing or is it a motor discharge?) In Cañada I like to search in the closets, I put order in my mother's closet, and I take some things I need. There is also a closet of my father and one which belongs to her brother. I gave my husband a shirt from my brother. Sometimes she takes things as this jacket she wears today. I also like to see photo albums.

Ana's thoughts go to a place where she gets things to meet her needs, and to put things in order. Again, one might wonder if this is her association with not getting what she needs from the analyst?

Analyst: What are you searching for in Cañada's closets? Perhaps a part of Ana, perhaps understanding the relationship with your father, perhaps understanding what happened to your brother?

Ana: (Silence, she breathes heavily, and she seems tired.) Friday, I had a dream. When I woke up, I remembered it and then I forgot it. Sometimes I even don't remember that I dreamed. There was that image of a woman that I knew then it erased, and I didn't know who she was, and that woman spoke of something that had disappeared. (Silence) Sometimes I think of my brother. I know he is dead, but sometimes I think he will come, that he could be alive.

Here Ana's silences are followed by associations. Again, she seems to be responding to the transference. The woman who speaks of something that disappears, and the wish that her dead analyst might come alive again and become the analyst who helped her get to this point of recognizing that her problems are in her mind.

What this last vignette points to is that with *certain silences* we need to wait to see where the patient's mind takes her. *It is what follows the silence that clarifies it.* Here is another example:

Lydia

Lydia is a 27-year-old physician, an attractive woman, who came to analysis with a life-long feeling that she never enjoyed herself. In the second year of her analysis, after cancelling the previous session, Lydia came into the session looking pale and exhausted. As soon as she lay down on the couch, she began trying to stem her runny nose with the multiple tissues she had brought with her. When Lydia could talk, she said she felt so "embarrassed". There was then a silence.

When Lydia talked again, she apologized profusely for cancelling the previous appointment. She then stopped talking, saying she felt anxious. She told me that she even had to cancel her appointments at the hospital, and then began berating herself for how she was such a "baby" about illness. She "explained" that she got up with this cold yesterday and was ready to go to work, when her coughing and sneezing convinced her this wouldn't be good for her patients. She thought about cancelling her appointment with me since she was so tired, and she thought it best that she rest. However, she couldn't rest because she was anxious. It was only when she realized she had a slightly elevated temperature that she called to cancel.

F.B.: It seems your embarrassed silence over cancelling yesterday's session came from your concern you were being a "baby". Only when you feared you might harm others could you take care of yourself.

Many of us might have guessed from the beginning of the session that Lydia's embarrassment and silence had to do with the missed appointment, and maybe we would say something to this effect. However, this encourages a kind of thinking, that is, analysis as intuitive speculation, which ultimately is antithetical to the creation of a patient finding his own psychoanalytic mind. While the analyst's empathic intuition is central to his understanding, it needs to be used in a disciplined fashion to best help our patients in the goal of self-analysis. In my way of working, I try to help the analysand see that my understanding comes from listening to what is on her mind via her associations. Furthermore, the specification of her concerns over being a "baby" could only come from her associations.

A Historical Look at Silence on silence

There are two major trends in the international psychoanalytic community that have contributed to silence on silence.

To understand some of the basic differences in how analysts work with silence, it is useful to consider our different approaches to the unconscious and the best way to bring what is unconscious to preconscious representable form so that structure is increased. In doing this, it is helpful to go back over 80 years ago (1934), when two articles appeared consecutively in the *International Journal of Psychoanalysis* that expressed distinct views on what is mutative in psychoanalysis. These articles (Sterba, 1934; Strachey, 1934) set a course for different methods of analyzing that still reverberate in current practice. It led to a chasm in what analysts interpret and why that for many years we hadn't been able to overcome. Thus, for approximately the first 40 years after Freud's death, there was a split in how we understood how deeply interpretations needed to penetrate the unconscious. While most psychoanalysts agreed that uncovering unconscious derivatives that push analysands into ongoing conflicts and enactments is a *sine quo non* of the psychoanalytic method, there are major differences in how understanding this helps patients get better. There are those analysts who believe it is only via the patient's *experience of direct interpretations of split-off unconscious elements that led to significant changes* (Strachey), while other analysts held to the view that it is *only by clearing the way for unconscious elements to become less frightening* will the patient be able to understand and accept how her unconscious rules her (Sterba). As I've noted, the seeds for this controversy go back to Freud's ambivalence over his move from the Topographic to the Structural Theory, and the shift from his first to second theory of anxiety (Freud, 1923, 1926).

The basic differences between Strachey and Sterba can be characterized in the following manner:

As noted above, Strachey saw the patient's *experience* of the *unconscious in the transference as the mutative experience.* He stated it this way,

Every mutative interpretation must be emotionally "immediate"; the patient must experience it as something actual. This requirement, that the interpretation must be "immediate," may be expressed in another way by saying that interpretations must always be directed to the "point of urgency." At any given moment, some particular *id-impulse* will be in activity; *this* is the impulse that is susceptible of mutative interpretation at that time, and no other one.

(p. 150)

But how could the patient directly experience the unconscious, which is unconscious for important reasons? Strachey's answer was that the patient would see the analyst as a more "beneficent auxiliary super-ego," in contrast to the patient's severe super-ego, and this allows the patient to become aware that "id-energy is directed toward an archaic phantasy object and not towards the real object" (p. 143).

In contrast to Strachey, Sterba saw *the ego as central to the change process in psychoanalysis*. He believed that change came about because of the development of a therapeutic split in the ego between the *experiencing* and *observing* ego. That is, the transference neurosis is worked through via the patient's increasing capacity to view his experience of the transference through what he calls the *dissociation in the ego* (i.e., where the patient's ego gradually develops the capacity for contemplation of his feelings and experience). According to Sterba, this allows the patient to recognize intellectually and render conscious the claims and the content of his unconsciousness and the associated affects. When that has been achieved, the synthetic function of the ego enables him to incorporate them and to secure their discharge. While overly intellectualized, what Sterba suggested was a forerunner of what became known as Ego Psychology based on the Structural Model. As suggested by Paniagua (2008),

The technique derived from Freud's structural theory is widely recognized as the most appropriate in the analysis of unconscious ego mechanisms. What seems to have been counterintuitive and is seldom acknowledged, at least in some psychoanalytic quarters, is that defense analysis is also superior as a method of exploring unconscious id contents.

Contrary to what is frequently assumed, drive derivatives manifest themselves in a more vivid way, calling for a technique more congruous with the structural theory than the topographical one.

(p. 222)

Although Freud (1923) shifted to the Structural Model in part because of *discovering unconscious resistances,* and depicted an unconscious ego in his 1923 and 1933 drawings of the Structural Model, Strachey, inexplicably, views *the ego as primarily conscious.* He states, "for the forces that are keeping up the repression, although they are to some extent unconscious, do not belong to the unconscious in the systematic sense; they are a part of the patient's ego, which is co-operating with us, and are thus more accessible" (p. 130).

To summarize:

1 Sterba believes that basic to the mutative process is a change in the ego that allows the unconscious impulses to be *experienced and observed.*
2 Strachey believes the cooperation of the ego is a given, and that the mutative process occurs via the patient's *experience* of the unconscious, acceptable primarily because of the analyst as an auxiliary superego.
3 Sterba follows the Structural Model and Freud's second theory of anxiety, while Strachey's position is closer to Freud's Topographic Model and his second theory of anxiety.

It is my understanding that the major reason we haven't viewed ruptured silences as significant moments to analyze is that much of the analytic world has followed the Strachey model, where the *interferences* in the patient's associations were viewed as less important than the *content* of the associations before and after the silence. However, it is my impression that as we have moved to an acknowledgment (to paraphrase Ferro) that there is not only an unconscious to be discovered, but a way of thinking to be developed, the recognition that silence can be an interference with the freedom to think leads one to a greater appreciation of the need to analyze this wish to stop thinking.

References

de Cortiñas, L.P. (2013) Transformations of Emotional Experience. *The International Journal of Psychoanalysis* 94(3):531–544.

Freud, S. (1923) The Ego and the Id. *S.E.* 19:12–68.

Freud, S. (1926) Inhibitions, Symptoms and Anxiety. *S.E.* 20:-175–176.

Freud, S. (1933) The Dissection of the Personality. *S.E.* 22:57–80.

Kraus, N. (2006) *The History of Love.* New York: Norton Press.

Levenson, E. (1988) The Pursuit of the Particular—On the Psychoanalytic Inquiry. *Contemporary Psychoanalysis* 24:1–16.

Paniagua, C. (2008) Id Analysis and Technical Approaches. *Psychoanalytic Quarterly* 77:219–250.

Sterba, R. (1934) The Fate of the Ego in Analytic Therapy. *International Journal of Psychoanalysis* 15:117–126.

Strachey, J. (1934) The Nature of the Therapeutic Action of Psycho-analysis. *International Journal of Psychoanalysis* 15:127–159.

9 Further Thoughts on Resistance Analysis and Their Clinical Consequences

I have written about resistances in analysis many times, and they remain as an object of my interest as there still seems to be so much confusion about how to analyze resistances. This chapter is an attempt to clarify further differences in how analysts' understand and work with resistances.

Resistances are ubiquitous throughout psychoanalytic treatment, and most psychoanalysts would agree that working through resistances is an important part of the curative process. As emphasized by Freud (1914),

> This *working through* of the resistances may in practice turn out to be an arduous task for the subject of the analysis and a trial of patience for the analyst. Nevertheless, it is a part of the work which effects the greatest changes in the patient, and which distinguishes analytic treatment from any kind of treatment by suggestion.
>
> (p. 155)

However, this "arduous task" that Freud pointed to often led analysts in the past (including Freud) to try to *overcome* rather than work through resistances (Busch, 1992, 1995, 2014; Gray, 1982, 1994; Paniagua, 2001, 2008[1]). Currently, there are various iterations of resistance analysis based on the following questions:

1. How do we define a resistance?
2. How much attention is paid to clarifying the resistance before interpreting its unconscious meaning?
3. How important is it to stay close to what is potentially preconscious in analyzing resistances?
4. How necessary is it to use the patient's own associations as a guideline for understanding the resistance, or as Donnet (2010) put it, how much do we "make the patient the active agent of the method" (p. 158)?
5. How necessary is it to include deep, unconscious meaning as a way of helping the patient work through resistances?

DOI: 10.4324/9781032658704-11

I will briefly discuss the first two points mentioned before elaborating on them later in the chapter. The remainder of the points will be covered in the two models presented below.

At its core, differences in defining resistances are based on whether one believes *unconscious resistances are put into place because the dread that drives them is based on the most primitive fears imaginable (e.g., castration, separation, disintegrating self-states, etc.).* Given such a view, one might believe considerable psychoanalytic work needs to be done to even bring the form of the resistances (i.e., how a resistance shows itself) to preconscious awareness in a way that doesn't arouse even more fears, and before the nature of the fears can be approached, let alone any unconscious fantasies that are driving the fears. The slow and steady work of analyzing resistances, their return, further analysis, their return, and so on is exemplified in what Weinshel (1984) described as *The Elevation of the Not So Good Hour,* where there is "an increased recognition of and attention to the less glamorous and exciting exchanges that take place daily at the interface of the analyst–analysand interaction, the more prosaic and quiet elements of that interaction, and the nuances of how the analyst and his interventions assist the patient's analytic efforts—instead of so much attention to those "frames" in the analytic work which feature the analyst in a starring role" (p. 89).

Another way to characterize differences amongst analysts is that some first analyze *how* the resistances occur and only slowly work toward the *why*, and others focus their interpretations on the *how* and *why* at the same time. These disparities can be viewed as based, in part, on what part of the mind we see resistances coming from, the analyst's view of how we reach what is unconscious, and how we understand the way patients begin to analyze a psychic event. The first view (analyzing the *how* first) is based on Freud's later discoveries of the unconscious ego, his second theory of anxiety, and the degree one views resistances as unconscious, stemming from the most frightening calamities in the patient's mind. The second model seems based on Freud's earlier model of the mind, where resistances were seen as being overcome rather than analyzed, and where Freud (1895) believed anxiety was due to dammed up libido, and that releasing this unconscious libido reduced anxiety.

While character defenses, like intellectualization and projection, are usually recognized and understood as resistances by most analysts, the *quieter* but no less important resistances that are enacted throughout every analysis have received less attention, even though there is a vast literature on this topic from the 1980s to the present. Tuckett (2019a) gives examples of these often-overlooked moments of resistance as "the impression the patient has been going round and round, silence, speeding up, hesitation, interruption" (p. 864). I would add sudden changes in affect or topics, the way the patient tells a dream or associates, or the myriad ways almost anything can become a resistance.

I will now present two models that capture the major ways resistances have tended to be approached.[2] As currently practiced, there are significant differences, but I believe there is a way to think of an amalgamation of these models, although theoretical differences might make it difficult. But first the differences:

Model One: In this model it is believed that we need to first clarify when a resistance is occurring in the *here and now* of the clinical moment (e.g., "I noticed that after talking excitedly about your date last night, your feelings seemed to darken, as if there was something troubling about these exciting thoughts"). The importance of working in the here and now is based on the principle that:

> In the midst of conflict a patient's thinking is very concrete. He can only see and think about what is immediately before his eyes (or ears). For long periods of time the patient is incapable of keeping a sequence of thoughts in mind while talking.[3]

Thus, the basic principles this model is founded upon is that to make contact with the unconscious in a way that doesn't raise excessive anxiety, it must be approached concretely and slowly through the preconscious. As stated by Green (1974):

> "the analyst uses the preconscious as a mediator and continues the analytical work towards the unconscious by following the route of communications from the preconscious to the conscious, aware of trying to reach the unconscious by this well-worn path, in which case resistances will slowly give way, inflicting the ego with only minor traumas".
>
> (p. 415)

Thus, clarifying the resistance in the here and now is a first step to analyzing the terrors (e.g., feeling states) that fuel the resistance, and in this way, we *gradually* help the patient move toward recognizing the unconscious meanings behind his fears. The purpose of a clarification is to first draw attention[4] to a resistance occurring, and only later adding meaning. Clarification is the elaboration of a dynamic process in words as seen in the analysand's action in language in the here and now of the clinical moment. It is the beginning of a process of containment. Clarification is not a cognitive process, for without the analyst's empathic involvement with the analysand's emotional shadings, it will not have meaning for the patient. While Birksted-Breen (2009, 2012) noted the importance of *reverberation time* for the analyst to allow greater freedom of mind, the same is true for the patient, and thus resistance analysis requires a time of "digestion and transformation" (Birksted-Breen, 2012, p. 833) to be worked though. This echoed an early statement by Freud (1914) with regard to working through resistances:

> The analyst had merely forgotten that giving the resistance a name could not result in its immediate cessation. One must allow the patient time to become more conversant with this resistance with which he has now become acquainted, to work through it.
>
> (p. 15)

Model Two: In this view, the resistances themselves are understood (and treated) as closer to *consciousness*. This belief leads to the view that it is only by identifying the resistance, and then elaborating on its *unconscious meaning*, that one makes resistance interpretations *emotionally immediate* and *mutative*. This is most often done via interpretations of the transference. Given what seems to be the assumption of resistances being conscious, this method could be useful much later in an analysis when the patient is able to observe his associations.

Brief Comparison

The first approach (Model One) is based upon half a century of clinical thinking, primarily in the United States, where a new approach to working clinically with unconscious resistances was pioneered by the work of Paul Gray, and continued in my own work and in the papers of Paniagua and others.[5] It is based on Freud's Structural Model, the uncovering of unconscious resistances (Freud, 1923), the unconscious ego (Freud, 1923), the significance of the preconscious in our interventions (Freud, 1933), and his second theory of anxiety (Freud, 1926). As Paniagua (2008) stated, "the techniques derived from Freud's structural theory made possible a more reliable and naturalistic access to drive derivatives" (p. 219). The method is centered on working with resistances to increase freedom of associations and the capacity for self-observation as the basis for self-analysis, different than relying on an identification with the analyst. I will expound on these points later in this chapter and the method's current iteration over the last half-century.[6] Gray (1982) also added importantly:

> Freud's phrase, 'There is resistance to recovering resistances' could well refer to a ubiquitous reluctance to consider, perceive, and conceptualize—both to oneself and to one's analysand—the detailed workings of the ego in its defensive measure against specific drive derivatives.
>
> (p. 651)

The second approach (Model Two) is the one generally accepted by most analysts and has been understood as the basis for interpreting resistances. For these analysts, the method seems to have been successful for many years.[7] I haven't been able to find a specific reference for its use, although it seems based on Strachey's (1934) landmark paper on *mutative interpretations*. He believed that in order for an analysand to experience an interpretation as emotionally immediate, it needed to be at "the point of urgency" (p. 150).[8] *This meant interpreting an unconscious id derivative.* As mentioned, it seems based on Freud's (1895) first theory of anxiety, where symptoms were seen as due to dammed up libido, and freeing the repressed unconscious impulses was viewed as reducing anxiety. As Strachey noted, "At any given moment some particular id-impulse will be in activity; *this* is the impulse susceptible of mutative interpretation, *and no other one*" (p. 150, italics added).[9] Here we see the emphasis on the impulse and not the defense.

The Clinical/Theoretical Basis for Model One

There are three significant changes Freud made to his model of the mind that are the basis for my approach to analyzing resistances. The first is Freud's (1926) second theory of anxiety, where he saw "the ego as the sole seat of anxiety", leading to an important differentiation from his first theory. "Whereas the old view made it natural to suppose that anxiety arose from the libido belonging to the repressed instinctual impulses, the new one, on the contrary, made the ego the source of anxiety" (Freud, 1926, p. 161). A second factor in this model is Freud's (1923) discovery of an unconscious ego, and that the *unconscious ego* was *the source of unconscious resistances in analysis,* which he saw as the key to working through (Busch, 1993, 1995, 2007, 2013a, 2013b). Thus, there was now an *unconscious ego* as well as unconscious id. The third component of this model is Freud's appreciation for the significance of the preconscious in mental life (Busch, 2006, 2013). One could see this view beginning to be expressed in his paper on "Wild Analysis" (Freud, 1910).

> If knowledge about the unconscious were as important for the patient as people inexperienced in psycho-analysis imagine, listening to lectures or reading books would be enough to cure him. Such measures, however, have as much influence on the symptoms of nervous illness as a distribution of menu-cards in a time of famine has upon hunger … Since, however, psycho-analysis cannot dispense with giving this information, it lays down that this shall not be done before … the

patient must, through preparation, himself *have reached the neigh-borhood of what he has repressed.*

(pp. 225–226; italics added)

However, as documented by Paniagua (2001) and myself (1992), Freud struggled with holding to his later discoveries of analyzing resistances, and so did many who followed.

The modern era for analyzing resistances began with a paper by Gray (1982), when he states that

It has for some time been my conclusion, rightly or wrongly, that the way a considerable proportion of analysts listen to and perceive their data has, in certain significant respects, *not* evolved as I believe it would have if historically important concepts concerned with the defensive functions of the ego had been wholeheartedly allowed their place in the actual application of psychoanalytic technique.

(p. 622)

He pointed out that the standard explanation for the slow development of the inclusion of the ego in our understanding of psychoanalytic technique was that in the beginning of psychoanalysis there was primarily interest in repressed content, and that it took time to appreciate the nature of the ego and its complexity. He challenged this view, believing "there exists a universal *resistance* to truly assimilating certain concepts concerning the ego" (p. 623).

There is a vast documentation as to how these observations led to a way of analyzing resistances and a revised Freudian method of analysis that has a common ground with other perspectives (Busch, 2013, 2015). The basic premise is that the unconscious resistances are based on the most terrifying feelings known to mankind, and thus must be analyzed with caution so that they can be grasped by the preconscious ego. It is only with building representation of the resistances in the preconscious ego that these terrifying feelings can be approached. After a lengthy period of time spent clarifying the resistances and analyzing the specific fears that drive them, we gain glimpses of the underlying fantasies *via the patient's associations.* It is a method based on the patient's associations rather than *primarily* through the analyst's intuitive understanding, which, from an ethical position (Diamond, 2014), can only be verified via the analyst's associations. Let me now present certain ways of working with resistances that have evolved with the principles noted above.

1 Clarifying *breaks* in the patient's free associations: This is often the first step in analyzing resistances. One can easily observe those times when the patient is associating and there is a sudden

change in affect, silence,[10] or a switch to a different topic when the patient seems to be associating to something meaningful. It is at these times we can observe a potential resistance in the immediacy of the clinical moment, and it is the most useful time to point out a resistance, as it is a psychological event that has just happened in the here and now of the session. Paniagua (1991) helpfully described it as intervening at the *workable surface*. For example, a patient saying something negative about her mother for the first time briefly pauses, and then says, "but she really tried to do the best she could". I would say, "I noticed after you said something negative about your mother for the first time, you seemed to feel uncomfortable, and switched your thought about her to something more neutrally positive." Thus, I am pointing to the affect that set off danger signals, and then waiting to see what part (if any) of the danger the patient can associate to. I do not speculate as to what the unconscious meaning of her fear is at this point, waiting instead to see where the patient's associations go. From another perspective, Schafer (1983) noted,

> There are many moments in the course of an analysis when analysands seem to dangle unexpressed content before the analyst. These are moments when the analyst is tempted to say, for example, "You are angry," "You are excited," or "You are shamed." But if it is so obvious, why isn't the analysand simply saying so or showing unmistakably that it is so? To begin with, it is the hesitation, the obstructing, the resisting that counts. If the analyst bypasses this difficulty with a direct question or confrontation, the analysand is too likely to feel seduced, violated, or otherwise coerced by the analyst who has in fact, even if unwittingly, taken sides unemphatically. (p. 75)

2 Clarifying the *enacted* resistance expressed in language action (Busch, 2009, 2013, 2015). This is when a patient's language is without verbal representation and closer to action—that is, when words become more like concrete acts designed to bore, seduce, anger, and so on. McLaughlin (1991) described it as words becoming "acts, things—sticks and stones, hugs and holdings" (p. 598). The analyst often experiences the enacted resistance first as a countertransference, and it takes some working through on the analyst's part to understand it as a resistance.

Clinical Example

Model One

This is an example of the slow and steady work of resistance analysis, where clarifying a resistance leads to increased freedom of associations, followed by further resistances, and so on The patient eventually comes closer to an important fear in the transference, and we then see more resistances, and later a further elaboration. The patient has been in treatment for 3 years. I will add my thoughts and inner dialogue in italics.

Mr. L, a 45-year-old economist working for a non-profit environmental research organization, came to treatment feeling depressed over how inadequate he felt about himself in his job, and in his relationship with his wife and children. Although it seemed he had achieved a great deal, he couldn't feel like he had and was generally isolated from others.

When we began analysis, Mr. L was almost relentlessly self-critical. Over time we could understand this as a form of melancholia and a guilty response to the expression of any need. Eventually his mood lightened, allowing him to become more expansive. However, there remained a certain formality with me, and transference interpretations were greeted with polite agreement. This was often followed by discursive intellectual associations. After repeated working on this resistance, Mr. L began to realize it was the same distance he had to keep in every relationship. He could understand this intellectually but kept retreating from it.

Thursday

Mr. L had just come back from a high-powered conference feeling great. He presented a paper, which was highly praised, and was invited to give an important presentation the following year. He seemed eager to tell me about his experiences. This was different than his usual way of experiencing conferences, where he would come back feeling inadequate. Mr. L then realized he was reluctant to tell me of his ambivalence about leaving the conference a half-day early to return for our session, feeling that he shouldn't have any mixed emotions about returning. At first, given what a good time he was having at the meetings, I felt I could understand his feelings of ambivalence. However, although Mr. L recognized that his concerns were exaggerated, it seemed important for him to convey to me that he had been disrespectful of the treatment and me. I pointed this out and added that it felt as if Mr. L was inviting me to criticize him.

As Mr. L seemed close to being aware of what seemed to me to be a regressive retreat and turning passive to active, I felt I could simply clarify it by highlighting it for him. I also added what I thought was a motivation based upon earlier discoveries. Previously he uncovered the many times his accomplishments would be belittled by his mother. Although demeaning, it was a form of emotional attachment not always possible with his narcissistic mother.

Mr. L's associations went toward his meeting with an older man, Kevin. Mr. L laughed with recognition when he said, "He didn't remind me of you." As Mr. L recognized the denial, there seemed no reason to point it out. He was collaborating on an article with Kevin, and when Mr. L saw the first draft Kevin had prepared, he was disappointed. Mr. L sat down with him and rewrote the article, and Kevin seemed to be very pleased with the corrections. Mr. L left this topic quickly. After a while I suggested that he seemed to need to leave this topic quickly after having critical thoughts about this man who wasn't me.

In this resistance clarification, I believe I can add its relationship to the transference as Mr. L had already made this connection. It is a way of remaining close to what can become preconsciously available to the patient.

Occasionally, then, Mr. L would interrupt his narrative to talk about the end of our last session, before he left for the conference. He had become confused as to whether he had told me earlier that he would be attending it (he had). He knew he had, but in his mind, he was afraid he hadn't mentioned it. Again, he seemed to be searching for something I could criticize him about.

Here again we see a regressive retreat similar to what happened earlier in the session. As it was at the end of the session and I had already pointed it out, I didn't say anything.

Monday

As soon as Mr. L starts talking, I find my mind drifting to some phone calls I want to make between patients. Having seen a patient immediately before Mr. L without having this concern, I see how quickly I am "outside" the session. As I'm sifting through why I'm feeling this way, I catch that Mr. L is describing a similar process of being outside the immediacy of the session. He was saying, "I don't know where my head is this morning. You know how I like to come in early to just think about what we've been talking about. Today I found myself thinking about my next grant. It was a lot of fun."

Here Mr. L retreats from liking to be in the waiting rooms to re-connect with me to how much fun it was to think about work. However, I find myself caught up in a countertransference reaction. How was it fun, I wondered? I've never heard him talk about grant writing this way. Why am I feeling a push to ask him about this? Often when Mr. L says something obscure, it becomes clearer as he continues in the session. I can't tell at this point if my feeling that I want to question him is to get him more involved or get me more involved. I then realize this feeling of wanting to critically question him is something important, but briefly caught up in a countertransference not yet understood by me, I remained silent. It is only later that I wonder if my thought that I would question him critically would have been a repetition of his relationship with his mother.

He then said:

I wanted to think about what we talked about yesterday, but I kept returning to thinking about work. Isn't this what I always do, retreat into work? Part of the problem is, and I don't know why I couldn't say this before, that part of me wanted to stay at the conference.

Mr. L then starts talking about his ambivalence about *going* to the conference in the first place in obsessional detail.

Analyst: I wonder if you noticed the switch from talking about your ambivalence about *coming back* from the conference for your appointment with me, to ambivalence about *going* to the conference.

Here I make another clarification of an inhibiting defense—the sudden switch from talking about his ambivalence about coming back from the conference to his ambivalence about going.

Mr. L: Well, there were some things I wanted to go to on Thursday morning, but in fact I wanted to come back for *you*. I mean *me*. Wait, that slip is important.

Mr. L then goes back to the incident he talked about yesterday, his disappointment with Kevin's first draft of their collaboration; he tells me that Kevin wrote him what a pleasure it was to work with him. Mr. L then wondered, "Maybe he's just saying that. Is this what I'm afraid of? I'm thinking how much I enjoy working with him." (He goes into obsessional detail that I found difficult to remember, and I start to feel lethargic. Mr. L realizes he's drifting off and he's not sure what he's talking about anymore.) **Analyst:** There seemed to be two thoughts you drifted from. The slip returning for *me and* wondering whether you are afraid of how much you enjoy working with this man who "didn't" remind you of me.

Here Mr. L recognizes his resistance, and I bring him back to what may have triggered his talking in obsessional detail. I remind Mr. L of his specific associations, not what I hypothesize is their unconscious meaning. (My clarification seems to make Mr. L more anxious as he drifts, in an obsessional manner, to more incidents he's already told me. As Mr. L repeats a story of negotiations around money issues with his boss, I start to feel lethargic. When Mr. L briefly pauses, I say: "I don't know if you have this sense, but I feel like you've been telling me a number of incidents today that I think I've heard you talk about before in a similar way. This incident with your boss is one of those."

Mr. L: I've had that feeling a number of times during the session. I don't know why I didn't bring it up. (Pause) I'm thinking of something, which doesn't make sense yet. When I come in here and you're ready to deal with me as a man, I feel like I can't do that. I back away. When I would talk to an attractive woman at the conference, I couldn't keep my mind on what we were talking about, and I drifted to sexual thoughts. Then I would talk myself into saying, "Nothing is going to happen", and I could get back in conversation.

Analyst: It seems, then, it's your sexual thoughts and feelings that lead you to pull back from me.

An Interpretation Based on His Associations

Mr. L: (Pause) This is really embarrassing. (Pause) There are times when I feel we are both really into what I'm talking about, and I start to get excited, and I get afraid I'm going to have an erection. Maybe this is a normal feeling, but I just can't let it happen. (Mr. L then goes into another long story about a guy he worked with who described making a business deal as "a real boner".[11] He then starts another story about a guy from graduate school who would say something similar about exams. I find myself becoming lethargic again in the middle of the story, but at this point I see some connection.)

Analyst: I think what's happening right now captures something important. While you're relating stories about these other guys, you bring in a lot of details that take us *both* away from the immediacy of what you're talking about. It seems like in this way you keep us at some distance, uninterested and unexcited about what you're saying. It seems to be a way of feeling safe from getting too excited and getting an erection.

Here we have my interpretation of the defense enactment. In this, I point to the process that's going on—his talking in great detail—that leads us both to feel withdrawn. In this way, he retreats from the anxiety over getting excited with me and having an erection. Thus, one layer of the resistance is revealed.

Mr. L: Frankly, my own story was boring me. I started to feel freaked out by what I was talking about before. But, you know, here I am 48 years old and still dealing with these issues.

Analyst: Now you present yourself as a shmegege.[12]

Mr. L: I'm afraid I will jump into your arms.

In this session we see how clarifying resistances leads to increasing freedom of associations, and Mr. L's capacity to speak the fears behind his difficulties with closeness in the transferencethat is, getting too excited and having an erection.[13] *Importantly, also, I try to help Mr. L see that understanding comes from consulting his own mind (i.e., a basis for self-analysis), rather than the analyst telling him what's on his mind.*

Tuesday

Mr. L: I'm thinking about what we *should* talk about. I should focus on what we talked about yesterday. I know it's important, as I see it happening all the time. I'm talking with someone, and I start to feel like pulling back. I say to myself we're not going to have sex, and then I can get back into the conversation, and I feel so much more real. It took me a while to get back to thinking about it yesterday. I feel like I want to escape from it. I'm not sure what it is. It's still vague to me. I need to get to something concrete. *I too am starting to feel vague.*

Analyst: I wonder if, with your vagueness, you're pulling us back from your fears that having me too interested might lead you to feel excited and want to jump into my arms?

Here, again, I'm clarifying the enacted defense, and feel it's important to bring in the fear as he's already mentioned it.

Mr. L: (surprised) I completely blocked that part out. I knew there was something important I was missing. Now it's clear, the part about jumping into your arms.

Analyst: And getting an erection with me.

*Mr. L's thoughts then went to how he was closed off from other guys in his growing up. He remembered never playing sports with other guys or being capable of being intense with them. His thoughts then turned to his father, and how he never considered him a success. However, he then brought up times when his father's achievements led to articles in the big city newspapers where he lived. (Here we have the first hint of his father as not simply some dull guy, but someone who could be exciting.)***Mr. L:** How does this fit with here? This morning when I was driving over, I was thinking how glad I was I found you. How from the very beginning we really clicked. Incredible, you were the only guy I interviewed. That's not true. There was this other guy who I got some information about but decided not to see him. I thought coming here was perfect. Your office is so close, and I could come to appointments on the way to work.

Analyst: So, you start out thinking how we really clicked, but by the time you're finished, you came to see me because it was convenient. The exciting feelings get drained off.

Again, I'm clarifying the resistance to feeling excited.

Mr. L: Am I afraid of what will happen next? Is it a fear of sex? I'm always afraid I'm going to wreck things by saying something stupid. That's why I'm always thinking about coming in and making sure I did my analytic homework. How will I get you interested? (He laughs in recognition.) It seems like it's just the opposite. Something came up yesterday that's been on my mind, and I wanted to tell you, but it's embarrassing, and I don't know if I'm getting away from what we're talking about. I'm going to tell you anyway. It will be interesting to see how it's related. It has to do with making love to Lynn [his wife] yesterday. We had a really nice day on Sunday, and when we went to bed, I had the thought that I'd like to make love. I started to touch Lynn's body, and it felt really good. Then it started to seem like an effort, and I lost interest. (He then starts to become vague.)

Analyst: I wonder if it also sounds to you like you're starting to talk in vague terms. This happened after having sex on your mind, just like with Lynn.

Mr. L: I can see that now. I was avoiding telling you that soon after I met Lynn, we talked a lot about our past sexual experiences. I found a lot of her stories about sex with other men exciting. I felt left out a lot. I only had girlfriends, and she had different sexual partners.

Analyst: So, you feel your stories wouldn't be exciting. At this point it might feel safer.

Mr. L: I don't feel Lynn gets that excited when we have sex. I wish sometimes she could be more like Rachel (a previous girlfriend), who would love to have sex really often, and initiate it. But you know I was much younger. (He goes on to give various external reasons why he was not interested in sex so often now.)

Analyst: There was something about Rachel's sexual excitement that excited you, yet you just retreated from it. It reminds me of your fear of sexually exciting me by showing your excitement.

Mr. L: The plot thickens.

As the fear underlying the resistance becomes understood, we see a return of the resistance. Once this is clarified again, Mr. L can again approach the fear in a more direct manner. This fits well with Tuckett's (2019a) conceptualization of resistances in the context of free association as "link-making, rapid emotional consequences, then link breaking" (p. 863). I would add that in Mr. L's case, we see clarifications of the link-breaking leading to more links to the meaning of the resistance, then further link-breaking, and so on.

Model Two

Strachey's (1934) paper on the "mutative interpretation" posits many ideas that seem to serve as the basis for Model Two. In the later stages of the paper, Strachey equates a mutative interpretation with interpretations of id-impulses.

"Every mutative interpretation must be emotionally 'immediate'; the patient must experience it as something actual. This requirement, that the interpretation must be 'immediate', may be expressed in another way by saying that interpretations must always be directed to the 'point of urgency'. At any given moment some particular id-impulse will be in activity; *this* is the impulse that is susceptible of mutative interpretation at that time, and no other one" (p. 150, italics added).

Further he equates resistance analysis with Freud's work between 1912 and 1917, where resistances were to be "demolished" (p. 130). Strachey didn't see this as much of a problem since "the forces that are keeping up the repression, although they are to some extent unconscious, do not belong to the unconscious in the systematic sense;[14][15] they are a part of the patient's ego, which is co-operating with us, and are thus more accessible" (p. 130). *However, in Freud's second model of the mind, the ego is not co-operating at all.* While Strachey views suggestion as an important part of demolishing resistances, the most important element he suggested was the transference, and specifically the analyst as an "auxiliary super-ego" (p. 139). What Strachey seems to mean here is the analyst as a *benign* superego, where the nature of the analytic method (e.g., invitation to free association), and the analyst as not condemning, softens the patient's harsh superego, which can then more easily allow for the acceptance of what was previously unacceptable.

In short, in Strachey's view, resistances are shattered instead of being analyzed. Id-impulse interpretations are the coin of the realm because of their point of urgency and are readily accepted because of a cooperating ego and the analyst as a benign superego. It is a very different view than Model One.

In a part of Strachey's paper that may not have been so appreciated as it stands in contradiction to the implications of the rest of the paper, he endorses the principle of "minimal doses". He puts forward the idea that "It is, I think, a commonly agreed clinical fact that alterations in a patient under analysis appear almost always to be extremely gradual: we are inclined to suspect sudden and large changes as an indication that suggestive[16] rather than psycho-analytic processes are at work" (p. 144). He believed that

"if the quantity released is too large, the highly unstable state of equilibrium which enables the analyst to function as the patient's auxiliary superego is bound to be upset. The whole analytic situation will thus be imperiled, since it is only in virtue of the analyst's acting as auxiliary super-ego that these releases of id-energy can occur at all" (p. 140).

Although the reasons are very different, the principle of "moderate doses" is central to Model One.

Vignette—Model Two

I will be using material from Roth (2001) as I believe it demonstrates a way of working according to Model Two. Roth presents her clinical material to describe the validity of different types of transference interpretations. I will be using one session from her material to describe what I see as her way of working with defense mechanisms (i.e., resistances),[17] although she doesn't mention either in her paper. The patient is a 35-year-old woman.

Monday

She told me that she had spent the weekend working on the project—she had a difficult meeting with her staff who complained she didn't let them do their jobs: she redid the questionnaires, changed all the arrangements—in her words, "rewrote the script", in major ways. She had invited everyone to her country cottage for the weekend; she now thought this was a mistake as it had obviously made them envious, since they are mostly unemployed, and she has a lovely house. Her maid kept walking through, the children's nanny was there and the gardener. She said how difficult it must have been for these struggling people to have to observe all this.

Roth thought the patient's tone of voice and manner of speaking were striking and conveyed a very particular attitude; she was speaking, as the French say, *de haut en bas*. Roth thought she was taking her on a kind of tour of her lovely, rich, full life and that she was meant to be full of admiration and envy.

Briefly, Roth suggested to her that as she was describing her weekend, Roth thought she felt her (Roth) to be like the "struggling staff", enviously watching her with all she had. Roth said she thought her need for this kind of situation between them had been particularly provoked by her realization that she needed her analysis and therefore was going to have to pay her, and that her description of the weekend seemed to be her attempt to reverse what she might otherwise feel at the weekend: how determined she was that she be the enviable center of everything, and how awful it would be for her to have to know about Roth's centrality for her (pgs. 535–536).

It seems to me that everything Roth brings up is something very far from the patient's preconscious awareness, that is, the wish to make Roth the envious one as a defense against the patient's need for the analyst and thus the patient's need to pay her (which I found puzzling). I could see if one presumed the analyst's position as an auxiliary superego, and that resistances were easily removed, then one could assume that such an interpretation of unconscious defenses and wishes would be acceptable. However, the interpretation doesn't seem to fit with Strachey's view of "minimum doses".

The Complexity of Using Two Models[18]

The difficulty in keeping these diverse approaches in mind can be observed in two recent articles by Tuckett (2019a, 2019b), which I will discuss only from the perspective of analyzing resistance. Tuckett is remarkably open and typically clear and thoughtful about his struggles, especially in the first case, which helped in identifying the two-model problem.

In the case of Andrew (2019b), there is one moment when Tuckett starts to interpret in terms of Model One but finds himself going further and using Model Two. He courageously acknowledges an enactment that leads him to make him go further than he thought he would, leading to a construction of what the patient *couldn't talk about*. In the other two examples, it's my impression he mixes models, while seemingly not meaning to. In the first example, toward the end of a session, Tuckett reports,

> I had said firmly but with some trepidation,[19] that it seemed to me he was struggling with the idea I was making him feel in an uncomfortable bad temper and he was having difficulty complaining to me directly. Second, *to my surprise* I later added that I thought he saw me as someone out to interrupt him. I could recall that I linked this to his wider complaint that he feels prevented from finishing things and so can't meet his obligations—wondering if he feels he is promised things which then aren't delivered and that perhaps this has been his experience for a long time. (p. 1072, italics added)

Here we see that Tuckett, "rather than simply draw attention to the patient's struggles with his thoughts" (p. 1079), goes further by suggesting what the thoughts the patient was struggling with, and then "surprises" himself by going even further. He doesn't linger on the question of why he thought he made this "surprise" interpretation.

In the next session, Tuckett starts out to clarify a resistance, but then once again goes further, which upon reflection he sees as an enactment.

After a silence, "I said I wondered (expressing it as a question), if he was now silent because *his thoughts* were making him uncomfortable" (p. 1074). Tuckett then goes on to say, "Was he becoming angry with me now because I leave him to get on with it?" (p. 1074).

Tuckett then elaborates: "I now think what happened here was that I had stumbled into an enactment on my part.[20] Although my intention was simply to bring a moment of resistance to his attention, I did not leave it at that and instead made a construction—explaining why I thought it was uncomfortable." He goes on to say that his construction led to "a frustratingly progressive mismatch of suspicious non-communication, yawning and fidgeting" (p. 1074).

Tuckett believes his enactment was based on an overvalued idea. He doesn't say what he thinks that was, but I suspect the overvalued idea was his reliance on Model Two. Thus, here we see Tuckett start his intervention by clarifying the resistance as described in Model One. However, as he recognizes, something compels him to go beyond that to make a construction of an unconscious dynamic in the transference, as in Model Two.

In the next session, after the patient has associated for 15 minutes, he becomes hesitant. After pointing out that the patient became uncomfortable with his thoughts (Model One), there is a pause, and Tuckett adds, "perhaps it was making him feel sad and a bit lost". Thus, instead of seeing where the patient's association goes after pointing out his discomfort, Tuckett adds a speculation as to what the patient's feelings are that make him uncomfortable. Tuckett doesn't say here why he went further. We do not know what happened next, but Tuckett experienced a warm feeling from the patient at the end. Of course, this can mean many things.

In a discussion later in the paper, Tuckett only acknowledges the second enactment, but I believe his explanation relates to all three incidents I've noted. In the following, he comes closer to highlighting the importance of clarifying what can be accepted preconsciously, and then how he needed to distance himself by going further.

> Rather than restricting myself parsimoniously to notice the clear and sharable fact that he had begun to suffer conflicting thoughts about his experience, I distanced myself to offer "understanding". In other words, rather than draw attention to his struggle with his thoughts, with ideas prevented from becoming conscious, I translated the content of what I thought his unconscious conflicts were into an idea of my own." (p. 1079)

If we had Tuckett's thoughts on why he needed to distance himself, it might give us insight into the reasons so many are drawn to Model Two. To remain in a position of uncertainty is an ever-present complication for the analyst (see Feldman, 2013). It is far more comforting to believe we already understand. Paniagua (2001) labeled this push to go further as *"topographically inspired"* (p. 672). What he's referring to here is that in the Topographical Model, anxiety was seen as relieved by interpretation that broke through the dam of resistances. "Whereas the old view made it natural to suppose the anxiety arose from the libido belonging to the repressed instinctual impulses, the new one, on the contrary made the ego then source of anxiety" (Freud, 1926, p. 161).

In the case of Thomas, (Tuckett, 2019a) works primarily in the mode of Model Two, with no further commentary.

After about 20 minutes, the patient fell silent. Tuckett notes this as a resistance and says,

"You have stopped, and I think you are terrified to go on exploring how uncertain you feel here with me. It is so frightening, so petrifying, to be in that state and you feel desperate to be able to be certain: to feel all is well between us so nothing about me needs to be questioned" (p. 855).

What I find interesting in this interpretation is that after briefly noting the resistance, Tuckett interprets Thomas' fears that fuel the resistance, and then, as with Andrew, once again makes a construction of the unconscious meanings in the transference. Here again he is working according to Model Two.

In addition to the examples above, Tuckett presents his theory of resistance analysis (2019a). After precisely describing a series of what Gray called "breaks" in the patient's narrative (sudden silences, changes in affect, etc.) Tuckett presents the *crux* of the differences between Models One and Two. He explains, "thoughts creating conflicting feelings begin to become *noticeable*—usually with anxiety attached in some form or other" (p. 864, italics added). The main issue for me, here, is *noticeable by who, and in what part of the mind*. It becomes clear that Tuckett is talking about the patient being *consciously* aware of a resistance as seen in the following sentence: "arrival of the resistance is a pivotal moment in the session when patient and analyst become *conscious* of a common problem which might be said to *demand interpretation* in the fullest sense—requiring understanding and/or comment" (p. 864, first italics added). However, what I've been describing in Model One is analyzing *unconscious resistances marshalled by the unconscious ego*. Due to the fact that we are dealing with an unconscious process driven by unconscious fears, the patient is *not conscious* of the resistances, and thus these must be approached gradually. If resistances are unconscious, it follows that it would take a fairly long period of analysis before they become conscious. As one might expect, for a long time, evidence of unconscious resistances are explained away or corrected by the patient. What Tuckett is describing, I think, is *how one can analyze a resistance much later in analysis, when a patient is capable of observing his own associations.*

It is not surprising that Tuckett only mentions two papers by Freud (1912, 1913) in his description of resistances, and leaves out references to Freud's later works, which set the stage for understanding unconscious resistances. As he seems to discount the literature leading to Model One, he erroneously states that it (resistance analysis) became "detached from the specific context of the process of free association"(p. 863), while indeed Model One is based entirely on the method of free association. Model One is based upon the analyst's capacity to listen polyphonically, which includes following closely the patient's association, listening to the patient's association as a dream, and listening for one's countertransferences and reveries and the associations that help us understand them.

Uncertainty and Model Two

In addition to any theoretical reason for the analyst's being drawn to interpret unconscious factors for a resistance before it has even become clear to the patient that a resistance has occurred, Feldman (2013) offers another possibility, that is,*uncertainty.* "I have briefly alluded to the disturbing and uncomfortable impact of the experience of uncertainty, helplessness, fear, or confusion in the patient, and/or arising in the analyst himself" (p. 54). Might it be that by giving in-depth explanations we are reassuring the patient and ourselves that we understand what is occurring, as Tuckett needed to in his example. "Indeed, the *very fact* of being able to formulate an interpretation may relieve the analyst (and sometimes also the patient) of these desperate feelings of helplessness and panic associated with uncertainty" (p. 54). Feldman adds, "It is not at all difficult to see why there should be a pull toward the notion of a correct interpretation, a selected fact, or a confident formulation of the patient's history. In addition to the analyst's difficulty in tolerating uncertainty and confusion, we might add the analyst's narcissistic needs, or his unconscious need to turn to omniscient and omnipotent means of reparation" (p. 55).

Feldman presents a clinical example where the fear of not knowing is palpable, leading to the patient's explanations. Feldman is able to stay with this observable resistance and does not need to give further explanations.

The patient begins the session by describing her disturbed sleep the previous evening, which bothered her as she usually has no trouble sleeping, and then she gives several explanations for why this might be. Feldman eventually says,

"I thought not knowing was difficult and threatening to her" (p. 57). The patient continued, "When my husband asked me my sleep—the first thing that popped into my mind is restarting my analysis. I can manage when I've had a good night's sleep. I used to be able to manage." After an expectant pause, she said, "The thought of coming in here agitates me in the night. Knowing that I'm coming back, and then before very long you're going to be away again. I don't want to talk to my husband about that. That agitates me, because sleep is very important to me" (p. 56).

The patient then began to talk about her sister's medical problems and their complicated relationship. "She proceeded to give a complex, fluent narrative about Carol's past and current medical and psychological problems" (pp. 56–57).

"After another pause, my patient added that she did not know what would be happening next year, and that worried her. She then said, "It *isn't* this nameless dread, this thing I don't know."

There was then an uncomfortable atmosphere in the room: moments of coherent narrative were interspersed with what felt like a restless, troubled, and broken-up form of thinking and speaking.

Feldman then adds that this patient always found it extremely difficult not to know—not to have one or several explanations for whatever is happening or has happened, even if they sound rather formulaic. She often worked hard to anticipate what I was thinking and what I might say or do. It was important to engage me in discussion, debate, or argument, the content of which was usually less important than the sense of my emotional involvement with her.

Feldman then says to her that he thought it was particularly threatening for her not to be able to account for her restlessness and agitation the previous night. The patient then offered herself and her analyst several alternative "maybes," none of which carried much conviction. "I think to myself that she was hoping, nevertheless, that I would take up one of her suggestions. *Indeed, I felt an intense pressure to offer an interpretation or "explanation" that would provide her with something to engage with, to agree or disagree with, to criticize or reject*" (p. 57, italics added).

We see in this example how Feldman is able to contain the myriad feelings experienced by the patient when she is uncertain, and thus able to point to the resistance to these frightening feelings in a way that might be most observable by her. Although he feels the pull to give further explanations, he recognizes this would primarily bolster the patient's defensive need to know. Lengthy explanations of unconscious dynamics before the patient is even familiar with what is being explained can thus be seen, in part, as an attempt to reduce the anxiety of the patient and analyst. While being uncertain can be anxiety-provoking, I also find it freeing to not have to know so much before the patient can tell me more.

Integration

I view psychoanalysis as a gradual process of containment by which what was once feared is not so fearful, leading to an increasing openness to repressed feelings and fantasies. I see containment as the basis for working through resistances. We start this containment process by putting words to what is expressed in the action of resistances. We attempt to build representations as a way of helping the patient contain previously threatening thoughts and feelings so that he can move toward deeper levels of meanings. As noted by Lecours (2007), what is represented can build structure and enhance the ability to contain.

As we are dealing with unconscious fears sensed by an unconscious ego, our first task is to make these resistances available to preconscious thinking. We do this by clarifying in the here and now the way a resistance appears. It is pointing to this "before the eye" reality in the clinical moment that gives the patient the best chance of observing a resistance in action. It is concrete, it is what is happening, it is not a speculation about something else. It is only with repeated clarifications of the resistance in its various forms over some time that the fears begin to be contained.

Notes

1   This is just a sampling of this perspective and appears throughout the work of Busch and others.
2   There are, of course, more than two models for analyzing resistances. For example, Green (1974) believes that staying close to what is preconsciously available leads to the unconscious, but he doesn't specifically address resistances. This is a variation of Model One. In the United States, neither the self-psychologists nor the relational analysts address resistances.
3   The data on which this is based can be found in Busch (2009).
4   The idea of drawing attention to a dynamic process before trying to explain it has, I believe, not received enough interest. I first noted this in 2015, and as Dehaene (2020) explains, virtually no information can be retained "if it has not previously been amplified by attention and awareness" (p. 241).
5   Rather than citing over 50 references here, they will be added to the text when appropriate.
6   There were two early papers (Kaiser, 1934; Searl, 1936) that presaged what was to come 50 years later. Searl's was especially impressive as she stated, "The analysis of resistances seems to me, then, to imply the knowledge of 'what' is subservient to the understanding of 'why?' or 'why not?'; and close adherence to this simplifying principle can alone gradually bring clarity and order into confusing varieties of attempts to deal with the patient's material, and can ultimately give us a firm basis from which to proceed" (pp. 476–477). As I've noted previously (Busch, 1995), Searl published a number of papers from a Kleinian perspective before her 1936 paper. Schmideberg, Klein's daughter, discussed how Searl was hounded out of the British Institute by the Kleinians (King and Steiner, 1991).

7   In a critique of this view, Green believes that going directly from the conscious to the unconscious causes "a real narcissistic wound, *due to the method employed for interpreting, rather than to the content of the interpretation*. In this case, needless to say, the patient can react to this intrusion only in an unfavorable way—either by a protective denial of his inner space, or by complacently accepting a false self and without really believing in it, or, again, by building up a masochistic type of therapeutic alliance: "Give me more interpretations, rape me, hurt me, I like it". This leads to an erotization of the superego, cheating it of its own nature. The rule that one should *interpret as near as possible to the ego* is justified if one does not wish to foster the establishment of a cement block of resistances which characterizes the beginning of interminable analyses" (p. 415)

8   First noted by Klein (1932).

9   In the same *IJP* issue where Strachey's article was published, a paper by Sterba (1934) was re-published from the original German (1928) where he highlighted a different view: the necessity of considering the ego in moderating anxiety (Busch, 2013, 2015, 2016).

10 I have previously noted (Busch, 2014) how silence is often treated as an epiphenomenon rather than a break in associations. In these examples, it is the content of the patient's thoughts before and after the silence that is analyzed, rather than the silence itself.

11 A slang term for an erection.

12 I am not in the habit of using Yiddish terms with patients, so I was surprised when I used this word, which, loosely translated, means a buffoon or foolish person. My associations after the session led me to think of how Yiddish was the language my parents used when they didn't want me to understand something, which in my mind meant sex. In this way I seemed to be bringing the sexual issue back into the treatment in this complicated form, which both captures a retreat from and the presence of sexual thoughts.

13 Of course, this is not the result of the work in a single session, but a long-term process of analyzing various resistances and other aspects of his fear of getting close.

14 Of course, in Freud's later model of the mind, there were parts of the ego that were unconscious in the systematic sense.

15 It is not clear what Strachey means by these repressing forces that are somewhat unconscious.

16 This is puzzling as he views suggestion as one part of the mutative interpretation.

17 I understand defense mechanisms as certain characterological ways patients defend themselves, akin to the resistances that develop in the clinical moment as described above. They are both instituted by the unconscious ego. I may be mistaken, but it's my impression that those working within a Kleinian framework tend to interpret defense mechanisms rather than resistances, the latter usually being more observable.

18 In a review of an earlier version of this paper, the Editors suggested I might compare my method with Tuckett's.

19 It is a puzzling feeling Tuckett expresses, without elaboration. In commenting on what he said, Tuckett was struck that "making my remarks made feel unexpectedly that I had put my head up to be shot at" (p. 1072). It's not clear why he saw the patient as waiting to decapitate him.

20 This awkward sentence is how it appears in the article.

References

Birksted-Breen, D. (2009) Reverberation Time, Dreaming and the Capacity to Dream. *International Journal of Psychoanalysis* 90:35–51.

Birksted-Breen, D. (2012) Taking Time: The Tempo of Psychoanalysis. *International Journal of Psychoanalysis* 93(4):819–835.

Busch, F. (1992) Recurring Thoughts on Unconscious Ego Resistances. *Journal of the American Psychoanalytic Association* 40:1089–1115.

Busch, F. (1993) "In the Neighborhood": Aspects of a Good Interpretation and a "Developmental Lag" in Ego Psychology. *Journal of the American Psychoanalytic Association* 41:151–177.

Busch, F. (1995) *The Ego at the Center of Clinical Technique.* Northvale, NJ: Jason Aronson.

Busch, F. (2006) Countertransference in Defense Enactments. *Journal of the American Psychoanalytic Association* 54:67–85.

Busch F. (2007) 'I Noticed'. *International Journal of Psychoanalysis* 88(2):423–441.

Busch, F. (2009) 'Can You Push a Camel through the Eye of a Needle?' Reflections on how the Unconscious Speaks to us and its Clinical Implications. *International Journal of Psychoanalysis* 90(1):53–68.

Busch, F. (2013a) *Creating a Psychoanalytic Mind.* London: Routledge.

Busch, F. (2013b) The Emerging, Surprising Common Ground. *Scandinavian Psychoanalytic Review* 36:27–34.

Busch, F. (2014) Silence as a Disruption. Meetings of the European Psychoanalytic Federation. Turin, Italy, April.

Busch, F. (2015) Our Vital Profession. *International Journal of Psychoanalysis* 96:553–568.

Busch, F. (2016) Unraveling an Enigma. *Psychoanalytic Inquiry* 36:295–306.

Dehaene, S. (2020) *How we Learn.* New York: Viking.

Diamond, M.J. (2014) Analytic Mind Use and Interpsychic Communication: Driving Force in Analytic Technique, Pathway to Unconscious Mental Life. *Psychoanalytic Quarterly* 83:525–563.

Donnet, J.-L. (2010) From the Fundamental Rule to the Analyzing Situation. In Birksted-Breen, D. et al. (eds.), *Reading French Psychoanalysis.* London: Routledge.

Feldman, M. (2013) The Value of Uncertainty. *Psychoanalytic Quarterly* 82(1):51–61.

Freud, S. (1895) Studies in Hysteria. *S.E.* 2:1–252.

Freud, S. (1912) The Dynamics of Transference. In *The Standard Edition of the Complete Psychological Works of Sigmund Freud*, 12:97–108.

Freud, S. (1913) On Beginning the Treatment. In *The Standard Edition of the Complete Psychological Works of Sigmund Freud*, 12:121–144.

Freud, S. (1914) Remembering, Repeating and Working-Through. In *The Standard Edition of the Complete Psychological Works of Sigmund Freud*, 12:145–156.

Freud S. (1923) *The Ego and the id. S.E.* 19.

Freud, S. (1926) *Inhibitions, Symptoms and Anxiety. S.E.* 20.

Freud S. (1933) Lecture XXXI: The Dissection of the Psychical Personality. *S.E.* 22:57–80.

Gray, P. (1982) "Developmental Lag" in the Evolution of Technique for Psychoanalysis of Neurotic Conflict. *International Journal of Psychoanalysis* 30:621–655.

Gray, P. (1994) *The Ego and Analysis of Defense.* Northville, NJ: Aronson Press.

Green, A. (1974) Surface Analysis, Deep Analysis (The Role of the Preconscious in Psychoanalytical Technique). *International Review of Psychoanalysis* 1:415–423.

Green, A. (1975) The Analyst, Symbolization and Absence in the Analytic Setting (On Changes in Analytic Practice and Analytic Experience)—*In Memory of D. W. Winnicott. International Journal of Psychoanalysis* 56:1–22.

Kaiser, H. (1934) Problems of Technique. In Bergmann, M.S. and Hartman, F.R. (eds.), *The Evolution of Psychoanalytic Technique*, 383–413. New York: Columbia University Press, 1976.

King, P. & Steiner, R. *The Freud-Klein Controversies.* London: Routledge.

Klein, M. (1932) The Psycho-Analysis of Children. *International Psycho-Analytical Library* 22:1–379. London: The Hogarth Press.

Lecours, S. (2007) Supportive Interventions and Nonsymbolic Mental Functioning. *International Journal of Psychoanalysis* 88:895–915.

McLaughlin, J. T. (1991) Clinical and Theoretical Aspects of Enactment. *Journal of the American Psychoanalytic Association* 39:595–614.

Paniagua, C. (1991) Patient's Surface, Clinical Surface, and Workable Surface. *Journal of the American Psychoanalytic Association* 39:669–685.

Paniagua, C. (2001) The Attraction of Topographical Technique. *International Journal of Psychoanalysis* 82:671–684.

Paniagua, C. (2008) Id Analysis and Technical Approaches. *Psychoanalytic Quarterly* 77(1):219–250.

Roth, P. (2001) Mapping The Landscape: Levels of Transference Interpretation. *International Journal of Psychoanalysis* 82:533–543.

Searl, M. N. (1936) Some Queries on Principles of Technique. *International Journal of Psychoanalysis* 17:471–493.

Shafer, R. (1983). *The Analytic Attitude.* London: Routledge.

Sterba, R. (1934) The Fate of the Ego in Analytic Therapy. *International Journal of Psychoanalysis* 15:117–126.

Strachey, J. (1934) The Nature of the Therapeutic Action of Psychoanalysis. *International Journal of Psychoanalysis* 15:127–159.

Tuckett, D. (2019a) Transference and Transference Interpretations Revisited: Why a Parsimonious Model of Practice Might be Useful. *International Journal of Psychoanalysis* 100: 852–876.

Tuckett, D. (2019b) Ideas Prevented from Becoming Conscious: On Freud's Unconscious and the Theory of Psychoanalytic Technique. *International Journal of Psychoanalysis* 100:1068–1083.

Weinshel, E.M. (1984) Some Observations on the Psychoanalytic Process. *Psychoanalytic Quarterly* 53:63–92.

10 The Memory Keeper

This is a story about a relational component of psychoanalysis that I've not seen in the literature but seems crucial with certain cases. At the same time, it is something that needs to be worked through as part of termination, when it can also take on other meanings that might go unnoticed earlier in the treatment.

Meeting my best friend from high school for our annual dinner, we quickly returned to our old roles, with the familiar phrases and jokes that sustained us through those turbulent years, and beyond. No one else remembered Bernie Schlossberg the way I did, or what it was like returning on the subway late at night from our dates with the twins from Brooklyn. Meeting later in life, without a plan, we would always spend the first part of our evening spontaneously remembering these times from the past, before getting down to catching up on our current lives, along with politics, movies, and jazz. I only realized later that these latter conversations were also a continuation of our past, as we formed our friendship around our exalted views of ourselves as "intellectuals", apart from our less thoughtful group of friends. The evenings we spent were enjoyable, but I always felt a little *melancholic* at the end of the evening. No one knew me at such an important time of my life like my friend. I found myself musing on this issue, and related psychoanalytic questions, that I hope will open a window to what I think is a unique psychoanalytic experience for our patients, and a specific issue it raises during termination.

What is uniquely psychoanalytic that keeps patients in analysis, and what makes it difficult, at times, for them to leave? While there are obviously many factors, a recent experience during the termination of a "good enough" analysis, like the dinner with my high school friend, *alerted me to the extraordinary power of the analyst as the keeper of the patient's memories.* It led me to remember a phenomenon I noticed over the years, but never really conceptualized. *That is, I find that when a patient returns after a number of years for a brief consultation, they will begin talking with the expectation that I will remember the full cast of characters from their analysis, as well as the key experiences that shaped them and how they were understood.* It is expected, usually correctly, that I have kept most of these people and memories

DOI: 10.4324/9781032658704-12

alive in my mind. In a good-enough analysis, the patient experiences the analyst as accepting of the patient's world as he experienced it, and the patient is generally able to accept the analyst's understanding of this world as told to him by the patient. That is, we mainly see and keep these memories first through the *patient's eyes*. When the patient is ready to think about another perspective, he will let us know. Ultimately, we open the possibility for new perspectives by understanding the multitude of factors that led the patient to this way of remembering.

Memories might change or be understood differently, parts might be added or dropped out, but they are ultimately understood and remembered by the analyst through the prism of the patient's perspective.[1] It is a unique perspective, as most of those who participated in the patient's experiences usually have their own version of what happened. I'm not trying to make a case here for the analyst as only an objective recorder of events. However, I believe we have to try as best we can to see and experience the patient's perspective in order to see the world she lived in and lives in, and how it affects her. Only over time might we begin to help the patient see that the way she ended up experiencing the world was determined by a multitude of factors.

Rarely do other people keep the *patient's perspective* on her experience in mind. In short, it isn't only that the analyst remembers the memories and characters in the patient's history; he remembers *the patient's mind*. Maybe even more importantly, *the analyst is the memory keeper of the patient's mind,* her unique experience of the world, how she has come to understand this world, and *how it has shaped her and she has shaped it.*

While the analyst as *memory keeper* is significant in its own right, it is especially meaningful for those whose experience of the realities of their existence were denied or questioned. For example, a woman with an alcoholic father remembered, as a youngster, seeing her father sneaking into the liquor cabinet and drinking a glass of scotch before breakfast. When she asked him what he was doing, he said he was "taking his morning medicine". While an apt metaphor from the father's perspective, it also denied his daughter's perception of what was actually happening. It captured the demand by both her mother and her father to deny that her father was an alcoholic and led to a life-long tentativeness in living her perceptions. Obvious signs of her husband's affair or her daughter's drug habit were not available to her. She literally couldn't believe what was before her eyes. For the analyst to take her perceptions seriously as something to think about and remember was at first terrifying, and later exhilarating.

Patients growing up with a borderline parent have the experience of continually doubting the veracity of their experiences. It's a matter of survival. The parent's hateful side is split off, and no one confronts this split so that the parent doesn't fly into a rage, resulting in the lack of confirmation of the child's perceptions.

A Clinical Example

Peter was trying to terminate a successful analysis. He had conquered the crippling anxiety and guilt that led to the panic attacks and self-sabotage that were wrecking his career. Consciously he felt the analysis was so interesting that he would like it to go on forever, but he also felt that he was so much freer in what he could do there were many ways he could use the time that analysis took up. Within the analysis I noted that while opening his mind to what was previously unthinkable (i.e., termination), Peter was still somewhat constricted in the capacity to reflect on his thoughts. He would leave it to me to keep in mind his thoughts and put them together, so that I was the interpreter of his experiences. *He had been much better at this before he broached the issue of termination.* Also, a particular enactment occurred more frequently once Peter brought up termination. At the beginning of a session, Peter would remember what we talked about the previous session, which often seemed at a distance from what I thought was most emotionally meaningful during the session. I realize that a patient's memory of what, to the analyst, seems like a minor moment in a previous session can alert us to a nuance in the patient's experience we haven't understood. However, this happened so frequently during the termination phase with Peter that it seemed like something else might be occurring. Further, at these times I often had a countertransference reaction of briefly feeling confused and wondered whether I misremembered the session. This experience and what it meant, along with Peter's regression from interpreting his own experiences, alerted me to some important issues that remained to be explored.

Historically, Peter was one of the patients whose experiences were denied. On an every-day basis there was the split between his private and public mother. At home, she was prone to burst into rage at the slightest misdeed of Peter or his brother, while other family members or friends saw her as accepting and sweet. She was the favorite aunt of many of his cousins.

When Peter was around 15, his father left, and his mother slid into a psychotic depression, and eventually was hospitalized for a short period. Peter and his brother never talked about this, and Peter's aunts and uncles were more concerned about his mother. No one spoke to him about *his feelings* after his father left and his mother's psychosis. Thus, life went on as if nothing had happened. The pattern continued when his mother returned home, where she continued to struggle with manic-depressive states. For most of his life, Peter was ashamed to talk with anyone about what had occurred.

My beginning understanding of the importance of the analyst as a *memory keeper* and its role in the reluctance to terminate occurred in the following session, after a long holiday weekend break.

Peter began the session talking about the panic he was in over a holiday weekend, which was very unusual at this time. He went on to describe how he was going away on Friday, and right before leaving he noticed that he couldn't turn on the sump pump in his basement. He had installed it the previous year to keep his basement dry. He checked the weather to see if there was rain in the forecast, and there was none, but he couldn't get over the panicky feeling that the sump pump had to be working. He knew something was going on but was too panicky to think about it. He had to get someone to fix it, although it was a Friday evening. He kept going through a cascading series of thoughts about potential disasters if the sump pump wasn't working, beginning with a flooded basement leading to the rotting of the wood supports for his aging home, eventually leading to the entire house falling down. His wife, who he often used as a sounding board for his thoughts, tried to calm him down, but no luck. Finally, he found someone to repair the sump pump, and when the repairman arrived and brushed some dust away, the sump pump started up immediately. Peter was immediately relieved, spent the rest of the weekend in a good mood, and had a productive period at work the day I saw him. He still hadn't been able to think much as to why he was so panicky. However, while he was talking, he thought maybe it had something to do with us, but he wasn't sure in what way.

I was thinking that this panicky feeling over something broken that would cause everything to fall apart had to do with the long weekend and the fears of what might occur to Peter with termination, which was in the background. However, this seemed too generic and didn't capture the confusion in the transference–countertransference, so I waited.

Peter's thoughts then turned to a question that plagued him throughout the weekend: Did the sump pump really not start when he first tried it, or did he imagine it?

Peter then had thoughts that seemed related to termination, but he showed little reflective capacity at this time, and the thoughts seemed to be reported in an emotionally distant fashion. He told a story of getting a prestigious award, but it was explained in such a way that I was having difficulty figuring out what he was talking about (*again, I was confused*). He mentioned a fellow in his division who people were trying to get rid of and how it would free up money for other projects. His thoughts then went to a co-worker who came to talk about a problem he was having, which Peter felt interfered with his own work.

Once again, I thought of connecting these ideas to termination, or of highlighting the lack of interest in the psychological meanings of these thoughts, but again I thought there was something significant communicated that I had been experiencing in countertransference confusion that related to Peter's confusion about whether the sump pump not starting was real or imagined.

At a certain point, Peter noted how distant he felt from his thoughts and their meaning. It was so different than how he was used to talking here recently, where everything had meaning. Peter's thoughts then went back to the sump pump, and he wondered again if he had really tried to start it and it didn't, or whether he imagined it.

(As this seemed to capture the transference–countertransference, I simply noted that this question kept recurring. It seemed important.)

Peter's response was that he knew he had tried to turn it on, and it didn't, but he doubted himself. His thoughts went to the time when his mother went to the hospital: "I know she went but I keep thinking maybe I got it wrong. I remembered calling my uncle when my mother began to threaten suicide." Peter then wondered:

> Did I? I know I did but now I'm not sure. Was my brother there? My uncle, the police, and an ambulance arrived around the same time. It was pretty chaotic for a while, but nobody said anything to me about calling my uncle. So, did I?

I said, "So someone affirming your experience would have made it real". I left it as a metaphor for the past and/or the present.

There was a thoughtful pause.

During this time, I was musing on this question, "Did it happen or didn't it?" My thoughts also went to his depressed, "dead mother" and his panic that his home would be destroyed if he couldn't get the sump pump to turn on. The question of "Did he try to turn it on?" led me to think of its mixed meaning, that is, did he try hard enough to help his mother become "on" (rather than dead), and its sexual implications. I wondered if thoughts of terminating were arousing old fears of what would happen to his "home" when his mother was depressed or in the hospital, or when he had thoughts of turning his mother on.

Peter: I just thought of something that's never come to my mind in here. Folded away in one of the books in my office I keep a note from my mother about her hospitalization, and other things. In this note she tells us how much she loved us, and how badly she felt for how she was. I'd like to bring it in so you could read it.

FB: So, I could make it real?

Peter: You could tell me if it really happened. You could tell me what it meant. I tried to talk to my brother about it, but he didn't want to discuss it. Besides, his memories are different than mine. I think now of termination and how ready I feel, but also, I don't want to leave. I don't know why?

FB: I wonder if you tell us one reason why today. I've been a person who has helped you hold on to and validate your mind. You're not sure you can hold on to your own mind after we stop.

Peter: I'm thinking of Judy (a high school girlfriend he recently brought up) For 40 years now, whenever I'm in an airport, I imagine her seeing me. I'm always careful how I look, and I remember to stand up straight. That's funny, that's what my mother always said to me, "Stand up straight". So now I know who Judy was for me. He then thought about a soon to occur vacation near a spot where his family vacationed. He remembered a time when he was on vacation with his parents but couldn't remember where his brother was. In this memory his parents were very happy. "I remember being at a restaurant and feeling they were a couple". He suddenly wondered if he was remembering this accurately. He then said, "Was this the start of my doubting?"

So, I thought to myself, we come upon the other potential meaning of "doubting": the doubting of the Oedipal couple.

In the next session, and throughout termination, these themes continued. Peter started out talking about a meeting he had with his staff, where the former head of his department was present. He felt that this guy remained competitive with him, which was confirmed by other people at the meeting. Peter was pleased that he was able to tell this guy, who wanted Peter to take care of a departmental matter, "Why don't you see if you can take care of it, and if you need the Chair to step in I will." His thought after this was a line from a Mel Brooks movie,[2] "It's good to be the King." He was quiet for a while, and then said that he was thinking about this meeting, the people there, and how I (the analyst) "know" all of them. "Who else knows them like you do?" His thoughts then turned to getting home early yesterday, and how he was putting the finishing touches on this new short story he was writing. His wife came home, and immediately started talking about some incident that happened at work. "It really annoyed me. I just wanted to be thinking about doing my own work, and not thinking about what someone else has in mind."

Here I think we can see the patient's wish to hold on to his own mind, and another possible meaning of the analyst as the memory keeper, that is, a retreat from the patient's wish to be the KING, and all that implies.

A few weeks later this issue came up again. As he was talking about the ways in which he was so much freer to express his opinions and to know his own thoughts, and how much enjoyment he received from them, I noticed that his way of lying on the couch was different. He was gesticulating while talking with a lively voice. Then came what he called the "Taliban" fears where he felt he had to tell me that he wasn't going wild, and told me of a meeting with Howard, his previous co-chair, who was warning him about going slowly with some plans Peter had for the department. He was really pissed as he felt this competitive side of Howard, who had tried to keep him in check. He then mentioned that an evaluation of his department by an outside committee had commended him on what a great job he was doing. His thoughts then went to listening to the news on the way home from work and sitting down to read. His wife came home and wanted to talk. He just wanted to listen to the news and read but couldn't say this to his wife.

Analyst: Here's the dilemma you seem to face. You want to have your own mind, but you're afraid of what you'll do. Someone has to keep you in check, but when it happens you feel annoyed. I think this is the dilemma you face in terminating; while part of you probably wants to be left to your own thoughts now that you've re-found your mind, this arouses your wishes to be the KING followed by the Taliban fears of going wild and being punished.

So, the analyst as "memory keeper" is another one of those multi-layered phenomena we become aware of in psychoanalysis that makes our work so complicated, but also intriguing. What starts out as a crucial relational component of the transference, that is, the analyst's ability to keep the patient, his world, and his mind in mind, also is part of an internal conflict of claiming his own mind and the fears this leads to. Ultimately Peter felt comfortable enough to set his own termination date.

Notes

1 For effective treatment, it can only be this way. As Schlesinger (2003) noted, the best way to approach the treatment is from the salesman's credo, "the customer is always right".
2 Named with typical Mel Brooks modesty, *A History of the World, Part 1.*

Bibliography

Busch, F. (1995) *The Ego at the Center of Psychoanalytic Technique.* Northwood, NJ: Jason Aronson Press.
Busch, F. (1999) *Rethinking Clinical Technique.* Northwood, NJ: Jason Aronson Press.
Busch, F. (2006) Countertransference in Defense Enactments. *Journal of the American Psychoanalytic Association* 54:67–85.
Colman, W. (1991) Envy, Self-Esteem, and the Fear of Separateness. *British Journal of Psychotherapy* 7:356–367.
Feldman, M. (2007) Addressing Parts of the Self. *International Journal of Psychoanalysis* 88:371–386.

Gray, P. (1994) *The Ego and the Analysis of Defense.* Northwood, NJ: Jason Aronson Press.

May, U. (2022) We are Looking Deeper than Freud ... On the Departure from the Primacy of the Sexual in Berlin and London between 1920 and 1925. *International Journal of Psychoanalysis* 103:328–349.

Paniagua, C. (2001) The Attraction of Topographical Technique. *International Journal of Psychoanalysis* 82:671–684.

Schlesinger, H. (2003). *The Texture of Treatment. Hillsdale,* NJ: The Analytic Press.

Scorsese, M. (1976) *Taxi Driver.* Columbia Pictures.

11 Are You Talking to Me?

In Martin Scorsese's classic movie *Taxi Driver*, there is a scene which captures a clinical dilemma that we often face in psychoanalysis and that poses a *challenge for aggression as a drive*. I see thinking of aggression as a drive as potentially *closing off other narratives that are more experience-near*, which may open up the treatment to new vistas.

In the scene I'm thinking about, Robert De Niro, as the embattled taxi driver, practices his quick-draw technique with a gun hidden in the sleeve of his jacket. He has become increasingly psychotic, railing privately about the filth and scum that he sees all around him, and plans to kill a Presidential candidate after feeling humiliated by a beautiful campaign worker (Cybil Shepard) for this same candidate. After acquiring a cache of guns, he is practicing his quick-draw technique in his lonely room, and while looking over at what is suggested as his imagined antagonist, he says in a threatening way, "Are you talking to me?" While the intent of the scene is clear (an imagined confrontation[1] with an adversary), as there is no one else in the room, one might wonder who De Niro is actually talking to, that is, *the imagined other or himself.*

Throughout the movie, De Niro rails against the filth and scum he sees around him. One could imagine that the intensity of his feelings is a result of a projection of his inner world.[2] We see this enacted *after* he goes on a murderous rampage against a pimp and others whom he sees as enslaving a 12-year-old prostitute. After he's done with killing others, he turns the gun upon himself, and we hear the click indicating the gun has no more bullets. When the police come to the scene, De Niro turns to them, and with a maniacal smile on his face, makes a gun with his fingers as if to shoot himself while inviting the police officers to do the act. So, the killing rampage against others staves off, for a while, the real object who needs to be killed, that is, De Niro himself.

On the surface, the imagined adversary confronting De Niro is another person. However, given our knowledge of projection plus his subsequent action of attempting to kill himself, we can imagine that it is *his split-off inner view of himself as disgusting filth that needs to be killed off.* In fact, his main cultural activity is watching pornographic films, with no affect, which leads him to take the attractive campaign

DOI: 10.4324/9781032658704-13

worker to such a film on their first "date", leading her to realize she's made a big mistake. In short, his aggression is an attempt to ward off his view of himself as filth and to protect his own life for as long as he can.

The dilemma for the psychoanalyst is mirrored in the question of who De Niro was talking to and seems to occur especially when it appears that the patient may be expressing split-off aggression, most often first picked up by the analyst's countertransference. This is then frequently understood as projective identification. The tendency to interpret what the analyst experiences as the split-off aggression in the transference is frequently interpreted as attacks against the analyst or analysis. Obviously, there are occasions when such interpretations are especially important. However, I would like to explore another possibility, which is, at times, *what seems like aggression expressed toward the analyst may be the patient protecting a fragile sense of self.* That is, the patient is doing something to protect himself;he is talking primarily *for* himself, and not *to the analyst* at that particular clinical moment. It is my impression that we need to speak first to what the patient is doing *for or to himself before we interpret what he may be doing to the analyst.* If the patient becomes angry with the analyst after split-off aggression is interpreted, *it may be because the patient feels that his fragile sense of self has been attacked.* In this way, aggression directed outward is life-saving rather than destructive.

An example from Colman (1991) expresses this tendency to interpret what the patient is doing *to the analyst* while ignoring what the patient m*ay be doing for herself.* As described by Colman,

> The patient is emotionally detached. Sometimes she brings rich material to the sessions, especially dreams, but they are all conveyed with the same lack of affect. She clearly expects me to do all the work and give her the "answers" she is sure I possess because, as she says, "You've seen it all before". Whether I do or whether I don't offer comments and interpretations her response is always the same: "And *then?*" or "Well?" making me feel yet again frustrated and that I have somehow failed to deliver the goods. But, in fact, she is unable or unwilling to use anything I offer.
>
> Gradually I have come to see how unconsciously she enjoys my discomfort and is deliberately tantalizing me (perhaps as she once felt tantalized?). She needs to maintain her refusal to take anything in to keep at bay her intense feelings of emptiness and, hence, neediness. She perceives me as withholding the answers—i.e., tantalizing *her*—and because she cannot bear this, attacks my thinking so that I am frequently rendered as unable to think as she feels she is. All this creates a vicious circle since the more she refuses to take in,

the emptier she feels and the more withholding I appear to be, thus
stimulating further envious attacks.

(p. 359)

The reader will immediately notice that the analyst views all her feelings as foisted upon her by the patient. The patient's "refusal to take
anything in to keep at bay her intense feelings of emptiness, and hence
neediness" seems not to be considered as something the patient needs
to do for herself. In fact, Colman notes, "As a young child she would
frequently keep food in her mouth, refusing to swallow it, and on one
occasion was found one morning still to have the food in her mouth
from the previous evening" (ibid., p. 359). We see from an early age
there something going on with the patient about *taking things in*. To
assume the patient was doing something to others rather *than for herself* is to approach the patient from a particular theoretical perspective, where aggression is central. We see this further in the analyst's
understanding of the patient's reaction to an interpretation.[3]

> Quite early on in the therapy she dreamt that she left a bare room
> in which she and her baby had no clothes to wear and joined some
> children in a sweet shop which she associated with a shop near the
> Tavistock Centre. I made the obvious interpretation that she was
> hoping for a sweet from me. She responded immediately, blush-
> ing deeply and aghast, "How did you know that?" Thus, even in
> the one moment when she could actually acknowledge her need to
> be fed by me, she immediately wanted to get inside me and take
> over my capacity to know—in Kleinian terms, to possess the breast
> herself.
>
> (p. 359)

Here again we see Colman interpreting the patient's reaction as an
aggressive attack against her, while the patient's feeling "aghast" and
"blushing", which might help the patient understand what it means to
take in an interpretation from the analyst, is bypassed.

Another Perspective

Hannah was a 35-year-old married teacher when she came for analysis. While she felt she would have eventually come on her own, the
immediate precipitant was that the headmaster of the school where
she taught told her he received complaints that she seemed increasingly dour in the classroom and lifeless in her teaching. Her husband
also complained about her behavior. Soon after we began analysis, I
experienced something similar, in that I struggled to find something
interesting in what she was saying, and I would drift off to think of

mundane tasks. Mostly, Hannah talked about the concrete details of her life, focusing on how people weren't nice to her. During this time, she rarely had a spontaneous thought that might help us understand something new about what she was talking about. In fact, her way of talking seemed designed to prevent such an occurrence. This wasn't a conscious decision, and from Hannah's perspective, she was saying what came to mind. Thus, it was a puzzle how to make of this way of being that irritated people, including her analyst, to preconscious awareness.

It wasn't clear to me what Hannah's way of talking and my countertransference reaction was about, so I would listen to her stories of being treated badly, and empathize with her reaction when, indeed, it seemed she wasn't being treated well, while keeping my empathy with her abusers to myself; that is, I would *think about* interpreting (in some form) how her way of talking led me to lose interest in what she was saying but realized this would be experienced by Hannah as a criticism, and that once again she would be treated badly. Was this her intent? As with Colman's patient, "was she frustrating me" to draw an attack? Yet, I have noted previously (Busch, 2006) how *defensive enactments* often lead to the analyst countertransference reaction of irritation. I was unclear which of these possible explanations was operating at this time, so I waited.

After about a year in treatment, Hannah began to show a livelier side of herself. At times she smiled when greeting me and talked in a more animated fashion. In one session, immediately after she was able to express her vivacious side, Hannah withdrew and began talking in her dull voice. Bringing this defensive withdrawal to her attention led Hannah to say, in an irritated voice, that she was "just saying what came to mind". I said I thought I heard irritation in her voice,[4] and wondered if she did also.

Hannah was able to acknowledge that she did hear the irritation in her voice, and after a brief silence mentioned that an image came to mind that she couldn't place. She then remembered that the image was from a movie where a woman's liveliness was confused with flirtation leading to a rape.

We could then see how showing me her vivacious side brought up a fantasy that I would rape her, leading to her retreating to her "dull" self. However, there was also the possibility that it was intended as an unconscious invitation to symbolically rape her by becoming aggressively critical of her.

The question at the heart of this chapter is this: Who was Hannah "talking" to, herself or the analyst, in her retreat from her lively side to her concrete and dull voice? While there is no definite answer, I would suggest that when the analyst observes a sudden switch in affect, like Hannah showed, it is wise to initially approach it from the side of the defense, as Freud first suggested as essential to the working through process. This is because if a patient is protecting against revealing a part of the self, *one needs to work through the reasons for the protection* before analyzing the unconscious fantasies. It has been well documented how rarely such an approach is taken (Busch 1995, 1999; Gray, 1994; Paniagua, 2001).

Up until this time, Hannah had said little about her life until she left for college, except that it was "pretty normal". Over time it emerged that her parents were evangelical Christians, and that the punishment for evil deeds was never far from Hannah's mind. Even so, she managed to have a lively relationship with her father, who would become bland when the mother was around. It only emerged at a later time that her recent change in character at school occurred after she briefly became aware of an attraction to an adolescent boy in her class, leading to the emergence of the lifeless, dour Hannah.

Aggression as Primary

In Michael Feldman's (2007) otherwise illuminating article on addressing split-off parts of the self, he demonstrates the problem one can run into with a belief in aggression as a primary drive; that is, it tends to always lead to an interpretation of the patient's behavior as aggressive, which seems characteristic of many Kleinian analysts.

In his introduction to a clinical example, Feldman describes the patient's especially problematic relationship with his mother,

> where any communication of his needs or his distress would be met with something like "Yes, dear". On the other hand, he felt intruded upon by the projection of his mother's anxieties and disturbance into him, and he often struggled to distance himself from her. In the course of the analysis, he has gradually *gained a greater sense of his own mind, his own needs and his own personality.*
>
> (p. 374, italics added)

Feldman also reports that the patient had a tendency to take over an object's function. According to Feldman, the patient would do this in the sessions by taking over his language and interpretations in an excited fashion.

During the time prior to the reported session, the patient had missed a number of sessions and had come late to others. He explained that his missed sessions were a result of "efforts to express a greater sense of autonomy and not to be too compliant" (p. 375). According to Feldman, when the patient returned to analysis after two missed sessions,

He emphasized that, in his view, not coming to the sessions was not an attack on the analysis, but the expression of his not being able to cope he felt exhausted. There was a part of him that suffered as a result. And yet he did reproach himself, and he felt accused and blamed inside, which made him angry. He felt he couldn't help it, and he didn't feel responsible.

(p. 375)

In Feldman's understanding, he recognizes that the patient showed some insight, but he was using it in an *angry, defensive* way. He goes on to say that it was important for the patient "to repudiate any suggestion that he was actively involved in something *hostile and destructive* by coming late or by missing sessions" (p. 375).

Feldman continues:

As the analysis has proceeded, the patient has increasingly felt the need to try to create boundaries, to assert himself by not complying with the analyst's expectations or his interpretations. He seemed to feel that the only way he could assert himself and feel stronger was by engaging in vigorous disagreement. Paradoxically, his way of asserting his autonomy seemed to involve an almost total identification with a powerful, confident figure, engaged in a vigorous argument with someone weak and helpless reduced to making predictable, unhelpful accusatory remarks. In this powerful role, he felt protected not only from anxiety and guilt, but also from the view of the analyst as possessing knowledge and understanding different from his own, whose thoughts he might not be able to predict or control.

(p. 375)

Later on, Feldman reports:

In the session I am describing, after a short silence, the patient continued, "I don't want to do anything I'm supposed to do—including my project at work. Part of me hopes it's a good sign, something more rebellious is emerging, and I'm not so compliant". *Later in the session, he said that he actually felt very healthy at the moment, and indeed he sounded vigorous and alert.* He told me that his girlfriend had developed a minor physical ailment. They went together to a Chinese herbalist and have both been doing healthy things.

(p. 376, italics added)

There seemed to be enough signs in Feldman's observations that the patient's way of talking, his absences, and his seemingly oppositional behavior could have another meaning. Many analysts view the patient's capacity to identify with the analyst's functioning as a necessity for termination and that it might have been possible that the patient's way of talking reflected the beginning of such a process rather than a defense. I was also struck that Feldman described his patient, at times, as insightful, and that he could see that when the patient "said that he actually felt very healthy at the moment" (p. 376) and that "indeed he sounded vigorous and alert" (p. 376). However, these signs were interpreted by Feldman not as growth, but defensive.[5] Also, it seems possible that missing sessions could have been the patient's only way of showing autonomy, however ambivalently. That is, if the analyst keeps interpreting behavior one way (aggressive), and if the patient has a glimpse of another possible meaning that isn't being heard or at least acknowledged, might it be possible that he felt he could only assert the value of his own ideas (and his displeasure with the analyst's view of him) by missing sessions? This also seemed to represent the patient's ambivalence, as he probably surmised that Feldman would interpret his missing sessions as an aggressive act rather than a sign of his autonomy.

Some Final Thoughts

The question of who the patient is talking to is not an easy one to answer, especially when the analyst is feeling something like boredom, irritation, or tiredness. It is at these times that many analysts believe the patient is doing something to him. This is especially true when the analyst views projective identification as a primary defense and is reinforced by Freud's move to his second drive theory, where self-preservation was replaced by the death drive, ultimately transformed into aggression. However, as I've indicated above, it is useful to consider that what is seemingly aggressive may well be self-protective, a matter of self-preservation. While De Niro murderously rails against the world in *Taxi Driver*, we see how it is an act of self-preservation; that is, it is his image of himself as filth that he unconsciously feels should be murdered.

Notes

1   I have written previously about the issue of confrontation (2016), where I considered it most applicable when a patient is using an action defense, especially when it results in a split-off wish. In such cases the patient will find it too unbearable to allow in this wish. It is with this type of action defense that the method of *confrontation* is most applicable (bearing in mind that the confrontation doesn't have to be "confrontational"). The technique requires arousing acceptable limits of anxiety around the split-off defensive behavior by emphasizing the disowned action. As long as the defense remains ego-syntonic, it can't be analyzed. Thus, I start the

analysis of the action defenses with a description of what the patient is doing when he or she is saying what comes to mind. By clear, empathic statements on what the patient is doing with his or her actions, we hope to bring back into operation a working ego.

2   The movie takes place in New York in the 1970s, where sex shops, porno-graphic films, and prostitution were ever-present in certain areas, and this is where we see De Niro driving his taxi most of the time. However, when he meets his fellow taxi drivers, they don't have the intense hostile feel-ings he does towards what they see on the street. Therefore, he is always distant from them. When he tries to tell an older, sympathetic taxi driver of his feelings, he cannot reveal this psychotic part of himself.

3   A recent article (May, 2022) documents how analysts in Berlin and London abandoned Freud's two-drive theory and focused on aggression as the primary drive.

4   An analyst-centered clarification. A variation on Steiner's analyst-cen-tered interpretation mentioned earlier.

5   I had the uncomfortable feeling reading Feldman's account, where he dis-missed most of the patient's ideas, that he might be enacting the mother's role of saying, "Yes, dear".

References

Busch, F. (1995) *The Ego at the Center of Psychoanalytic Technique.* Northwood, NJ: Jason Aronson Press.

Busch, F, (1999) *Rethinking Clinical Technique.* Northwood, NJ: Jason Aronson Press.

Colman, W. (1991) Envy, Self-Esteem and the Fear of Separateness. *British Journal of Psychotherapy* 7:356–367.

Feldman, M. (2007) Addressing Parts of the Self. *International Journal of Psychoanalysis* 88:371–386.

Gray, P. (1994) *The Ego and the Analysis of Defense.* Northwood, NJ: Jason Aronson Press.

May, U. (2022) We are Looking Deeper than Freud … On the Departure from the Primacy of the Sexual in Berlin and London between 1920 and 1925. *International Journal of Psychoanalysis* 103:328–349.

Paniagua, C. (2001) The Attraction of Topographical Technique. *International Journal of Psychoanalysis* 82:671–684.

12 The Dreamer Who Couldn't Dream Her Dreams

Since the early days of Freud, dreams and the work with dreams have always taken a special place in psychoanalysis. One of the most fascinating ways of looking at dreams is the use of symbols and what they may betray about the unconscious. This soon offered ample room for jokes and ridicule: sometimes a cigar is just a cigar. But dreams also reveal the mind at work. In particular, the work of secondary revision of a dream —how well a dream is formed— can show the clinician something about the ego's capacity to handle un- and preconscious material emerging in the dream content. Since these early days, much has been written about the understanding of dreams. What I will elaborate on in this chapter is a particular way of listening to and understanding dreams when they are in the form of language action.

M—The Patient

M is a patient who had extensive night dreams but was unable to dream her dreams. When reacting to her dreams, she mostly talked about her *feelings* within the dream but seemed unable to associate to the symbols in dreams even with prompting. One could put it that *she seemed unable to represent her dream representations or symbolize her symbols.* Further, this patient's way of talking was similar to that described by Green (2000) and left me with similar feelings; "it was a discourse that seemed to be kept at a distance, developed at length on the basis of generalities expressed in broken speech that gave me the impression I was looking for my way in the fog" (Green, 2000, p. 431). I will suggest that this patient's dreams weren't dreams in the Bionian sense but were more like *actions* as part of an *interpsychic* process (Bolognini, 2004). Diamond (2014) described it this way: "interpsychic refers to the analyst focusing on the intersection of two unconscious minds—two interacting psychic systems"(ibid., p. 542). M would often *want to luxuriate in the feelings she had in her dreams.* Thus, when awakened by her alarm clock, she often felt annoyed that she had to leave the dream.

DOI: 10.4324/9781032658704-14

Clinical Example

The patient, M, is a 45-year-old successful hospital administrator, an attractive woman, who came to see me because of her feeling that life was passing her by. She has been in analysis for 3 years. She had been married for 10 years and had one child. She initiated a divorce approximately 2 years before coming to see me. M reports her childhood as being a mixture of over-stimulation and neglect. From early on, she slept in her parents' bed and was frequently exposed to parental nudity, intercourse, and fighting, including some physical violence. M's mother is a successful lawyer and the major breadwinner in the family. M's father is described as charming, passive, ineffectual, and possibly psychotic at times.

The transference has been primarily a highly idealized one. In some fantasy of the "good patient", a conflict emerging in one session would be "solved" by the next. Approximately a year into the treatment, the patient started having vivid sexual fantasies about the two of us, leading to frequent masturbation and, according to her, her first orgasm through clitoral stimulation. My reaction to these fantasies was most often to feel *imposed* upon. This wasn't a common reaction I had when similar fantasies came up with different patients. At the time, I didn't have any associations with this feeling, which was unusual, so I waited to see what developed.

Also striking was an enacted transference, leading to a particular countertransference. M had a way of talking that often left me confused and irritable. For a long time, I felt puzzled by my reaction. As best as I can describe it, she would start a sentence, pause, seemingly start in the middle of the previously started sentence, and it would go on like this. As you will see, similar countertransference reactions of confusion and irritation were typical in the sessions that follow.

Session 1 (Monday)

The patient started the session by saying: "I had a dream the other night. We were in a room together that was right next to your kitchen. The door was open, and you walked out. After a while I figured I was supposed to leave, but my bag was in the kitchen where you were talking with your wife. My bag was a big messenger bag that was stuffed (puts her arms out wide to show me how big the bag was). So, I stayed in the room and there were two jewelry boxes. One was off to the side and there was this other one that was mine. It was very ornate, and it was filled with all kinds of jewelry. I was having a hard time getting it to close, but I finally did. Then I went over to listen at the door to the kitchen and I didn't hear voices, so I figured your wife had left. I went in and said to you, 'I left my bag' and you handed it to me and said, 'Thank you', and I said 'No, thank you'. The bag was filled almost to overflowing with your psychoanalytic papers. Then I went outside, and I saw Sara (her daughter) and a friend playing together. There was also a moving van, and two Swiss maids were loading all the furniture into it. I wondered why all the furniture was being moved from *my room*. The funny thing was it all looked like doll furniture. Then after all the furniture was packed up, I guessed I had to leave, so I got in the moving van with the two girls and started to drive. When I got out into the street I saw my car, so I stopped the van and walked back to my car. I was walking down the middle of the street and cars were swerving past me. It felt very dangerous, and I woke up."

I was struck by how many symbols in the dream seemed to relate to various wishes and conflicts we had been working on, and at first, I saw the dream as a confirmation of these themes. I had lots of associations as M told the dream. The first was to Freud's interpretation of Dora's jewel box as her genitals. Its ornateness led to my thinking of it being made attractive and special. The idea that it was stuffed, as was the bag she left in the kitchen, seemed related to her ongoing terror of having been castrated and her fantasy of having a penis, something we had discussed at length. M had googled me at some point and found out that my wife is a Swiss-trained psychoanalyst, who, in the dream, has now become a maid. There are also elements of the primal scene and the idea she had a room in my house, said without affect. I was reminded of a time earlier in treatment when I felt invaded by her finding out information about what I was doing and even the way she came into my office. Strikingly, I felt like I was thinking in a desert. I had all these ideas but there was no one to share them with. This seemed to match what M was feeling in the dream.

In a somewhat emotional tone of feeling hurt, M talked of *feeling lonely* in the dream, and wondered why she was kicked out. Then she was in this dangerous place and *felt* alone. She then went on to describe how *held* she *felt* in the relationship with me earlier in the treatment, and while that's still there, it's not the same, and she feels more alone. She goes on in this way for some time in a complaining fashion.

The dream seemed filled with sexual symbolism, yet M's associations with it struck me as about being cared about or not, with her as a victim. M had, up to this point, not been able to associate to dreams, but only talked about the feelings. I had wondered with her about this before without any further understanding. I realized at this point I had been interested in the symbolism in the dream, and I was feeling left out of her psychic life (like she was feeling left out in her association to the dream). I didn't realize at the time that her thought about being left out might have been an association to the dream, albeit in a different type of language.

FB: While I'm sure your feelings of being alone are related to the dream, I wonder if you can see how you've stayed away from the different elements in the dream. *(Defense interpretation)*
(M responds with a "Hmm", as if she finds that interesting, which is not atypical for her.)

M: I tried to think about the dream, but I just get caught up in the feelings of the dream. It seems like I can't get out of it, and I just feel that way all day.
I felt at the time like I was confused about what feelings she was referring to. I wondered then why I was confused, as it seemed clear she was referring to feelings she described as being left out. What this confusion was about seemed important, but no images or thoughts came to mind. The post-Bionians, especially Ogden, consider the analyst's inability to have reveries in response to a patient as a sign of the patient's lack of representative thought.

M: I did have one thought, but I don't think it's what you're thinking. I was reminded of playing with my grandmothers' jewelry boxes when I was a child. I would play for hours in dress-up games.
FB: You said you thought I'd be thinking something else.
M: I don't know what that would be but not that ... You know a lot of times I feel like a little girl with you, and feel like I have to protect myself. But there was one time last week when you were talking, and I found I could just listen. I wasn't feeling defensive, and it just felt so cool. I could really get what you were saying, and it felt amazing ... I did notice there were a lot of 2's in the dream—two Swiss maids, two girls, two jewelry boxes. But I couldn't think anything about them. I also thought my daughter in the dream represented me. Like maybe I was your daughter in the dream.

This was where this first session ended. I knew something important was going on, but I was in the dark as to what.

Session 2 (Tuesday)

During this session I became acutely aware of M's telegraphic ways of talking. That is, between words and the end of sentences, there were lots of dots and dashes. A typical example might be for her to begin, "So yesterday ... I mean—there was all this feeling—but then *IT* wasn't the same. I was relieved ... It was interesting ..."

At this point I was, once again, perplexed about what the "IT" was, but I suspected my feeling of confusion was an important part of what was going on. I started to feel irritated and wondered about it. A memory then came to mind of being around age 4, when our apartment was being renovated and for a period of about a month my family stayed in a hotel, and we all slept in one room. This association came to mind in my analysis when I was trying to understand my frustration with instructors who I felt were saying things that didn't make sense. So, my irritation with M seemed, at first look, a countertransference reaction to something going on that I was listening to but didn't understand. My association, and feeling, seemed to be a typical primal scene memory and experience. I then remembered that M was exposed to continual primal scene experiences. However, I still wasn't sure as to how what M was trying to communicate differentiated from what may have been my idiosyncratic reaction to it, so I waited.

I finally figured out the "it" M was referring to, which she remembered as coming from what she described as "*our* understanding of the dream", which revolved around her being drawn to feel like a victim. However, my memory was that there was no understanding from the dream, only *her feeling about the dream*, and I had a "huh!" reaction in my own mind. She felt after the session that *IT* (that word again) had come to such a *climax, and* she could breathe again. I thought of the sexual meaning of this word, *climax*, which M seemed to not have any awareness of. *My feeling was that there was something erotic going on here, but if I mentioned it M might acknowledge it, but not be able to do anything with it, like with the dream symbols. Again, I felt frustrated and wondered about my countertransference reaction, that is, there is something going on that is sexual, but I'm supposed to not say anything about it. I experienced M as saying in language action "You think you're seeing something, but it's nothing".*

The patient went on to talk about wanting something so much, but never being able to have it. *I think here she felt she was referring to me, but it was vague.* She then started talking about going into a store (it sounded like with her mother) and being told, "Get away from that, don't touch it, and having her hand slapped". *I wondered if what was being enacted was a psychoanalytic warning from the patient, "get away from that".*

After a brief pause, the patient started talking even more in this telegraphic fashion, where it was almost impossible to understand what she was referring to. As I got the gist, she seemed to be talking about her demanding work and the difficult people she has to work with. After a while of this, I said,

FB: I hear your words, but I find myself losing your meaning. Your sentences seem to start and stop mid-way, and then there's another thought that seems related, but I'm not clear how. Is this something you can see? (*This is my attempt to clarify language action. See Addendum B).*

M: Well, I didn't want to be talking about it. After I said what I started out with in the session, and you didn't say anything I figured OK, and this is what I thought of ... but it's not what I wanted to talk about. I feel there are all these people stacked up and I'm on the bottom of the pile. I don't want to bring them in here.

M: (a bit more belligerent) I felt like you might want me to talk about these other things, like how I get along with people at work, and the feelings they bring up, but that's your agenda. *(This surprised me as I didn't remember even thinking this is something she should be talking about.)* I feel it's intrusive like when you close the door loud. (Then tears.) I want the session to just be about you and me. I've never had a relationship where it's just about me.

I noticed that her wanting the session to be about "just you and me" became at the end "just about ME". I wondered if there was anything I might have pushed her to talk about, and I believe the one issue that she could have seen this way was when I asked her about the dream symbols. I believed at the time I was inviting her to think about the dream symbols, but given her adverse reaction, I could image how she felt pushed. M wanted to luxuriate in the dream.

Session 3 (Wednesday)

M: I'm in a strange place. I had another dream. *(Long pause.)* I don't know why I don't want to talk about other things. *(Long pause).* The dream was about you and me. I just wanted to stay in the dream and when my alarm clock went off it felt jarring. I don't know. I think when I come in and tell you how I understood and saw something you said, I feel like it's a gift. When you explain something to me, and I can really understand, it feels like such a gift, and I want to give something back. It's like the jewelry box in the dream, and how it was overflowing. That's what I feel you've given me. While I see how it could also be about something else, but that's not what it *felt* like. Then in the dream I tried to close the box, and I couldn't. *(Anxious laugh.)* But I finally did. It's like the messenger bag full of books. That's what you've given me *(i.e., this thirst and access to reading). (Long pause.)* I feel like I'm avoiding something. *(Long pause.)* You know when I told you my dreams earlier in the treatment, when they were so sexually explicit, I felt they were so forceful, I felt like I was forcing them on you, and I don't want to do that. I didn't think you liked it. (Long pause.) OK. *(Anxious laugh.)*

Here's the dream. We were in this beautiful room with large windows that looked out on this pastoral scene. There was a beautiful mahogany piece, a couch, or taller, more like a massage table. I was lying on the massage table, and you were behind me like usual. I realized you were having a phone session and saying something like, "you put your hand like this, and you touch here", and I realized you were talking about doing massage. I asked what you were doing, and you said, "You want to try it", and I said "sure". Then I said, "I guess your wife isn't here" and you reacted like it was no big deal. So, I turned over and you got on top of me and put your hand on my shoulder and I could feel your touch, but just barely. There was a gentle pressure that just felt wonderful. You had no clothes on, and when I was coming into the session, I realized I didn't have a bra on in the dream and wondered about that. *(Embarrassed laugh.)* Then things changed. Two young boys came running past the window and looked in. Then you put on your shirt and jacket then I got dressed. There was no discussion. It shifted then and I was cleaning your glasses, and you were cleaning mine. You made mine nice and clean but there was this hard stuff on your glasses, and I couldn't get it off. I think I bent them some.

I asked you, "Don't you think your wife will be mad?" You said, "I don't think so". Then I woke up. I didn't want to. I wanted to stay in the dream. It was like falling in love with you all over again, except this time it wasn't all about sex. I felt a little annoyed that I wanted to stay in the dream because I wanted to read some stuff, but I also wanted to stay in the dream.

I know there are these other parts of the dream, but I don't want to go there yet. It's like with you. I know I'm going to have to, and maybe want to find somebody who can meet all these needs, but I'm not ready to leave you yet.

Session 4

She started the session by saying that she had some thoughts about the dream from yesterday. She imagined the two boys were of different ages, and she thought of them as our children. In a subtly distasteful manner, she said they were being competitive. Then she thought about the glasses, and she was cleaning mine and I was cleaning hers. She looked over and saw that I was getting her glasses very clean, but she thought I was being rough with them and that I was bending the long piece that goes to the ear. She was cleaning my glasses, but there was this spot she couldn't get clean. M then started talking about how I keep bringing up this topic, which she agrees with, she gets it *(a little more irritation in her voice)*. She doesn't have a penis, there's nothing there, and thoughts like that, but there are other things she thinks about, like the dream yesterday.

FB: So, can we say the spot you couldn't get out is what you think of as my blind spot; that is, that I keep talking about this one thing.

After a brief pause, M gives an indication that I've said something she's thinking about with an "Hmm". She then starts thinking about this earpiece on her glasses, and wondered since it seemed bent, would it stick out? Yet when she put the glasses on, they fit perfectly, like a warm, comfortable glove. It was like the touching in the dream in the massage; it was so gentle, not rough.

From the beginning of the session, I saw a progression in M's capacity to dream her dreams, for example, starting the session with "I thought about the dream yesterday", and elaborating on the two boys and cleaning the glasses. Also, I re-discovered my mind and was able to have thoughts about her dream thoughts. This led me to think I might be able to begin clarifying and interpreting the way she dealt with dreams.

FB: Things seem to be different today in that you're able to have thoughts about your dream. Previously there seemed to be a lot of sexual symbolism in your dreams … my climbing on top of you without clothes, the glasses I fix for you that have this piece sticking out … but I had the impression that I was supposed to react like nothing was going on. I'm reminded of the time when you were exposed to a lot of parental nudity and sex, but people acted like nothing happened. I wonder if you are now putting me in the position of being the one exposed to all this sexual symbolism, and you are the one saying nothing like that is going on.

M: I can see that, but I just don't want it to be there. While I feel there has been this split, I think it's in the process of healing.

She goes on in a somewhat psychobabble-like manner. Then there is what seems like a thoughtful pause, after which she continues: "A few years ago, I tried to bring up with my mother all the sexual stuff I was exposed to. She denied anything like that happened, and I remember how frustrated I felt." M then put her hands over her face and said she was ashamed of her next thought. After a period of silence, she mentioned that when her son became an adolescent, he confronted her and her then husband about the way they walked around the house with few clothes on. She angrily denied it at first, but then had to agree he was right. She felt terrible.

(M's ability to associate to two memories, which hadn't come up before, made it seem like my interpretation was in her "neighborhood".)

Discussion

As early as 1914, Freud described how words could be used as actions. He states, the patient does not *remember* anything of what he has forgotten but *acts* it out. He reproduces it not as a memory but as an action; he *repeats* it, without, of course, knowing that he is repeating it.

However, for the most part, this aspect of Freud's insight tended to fade into the background in favor of an emphasis on the patient's verbal communications. More recently there are those from the relational and interpersonal schools who have claimed what seems to me to be clinically indefensible, that is, that all words are actions. My own view is that words are used in psychoanalysis on a continuum from actions to communications.

With regard to the clinical material itself, most often in analysis it is the convergence of multiple factors that leads one to a sense of conviction of what is occurring in the immediacy of the clinical moment. With M, it was primarily my countertransference reaction, and my associations to it, that led me to listen more carefully to the effect on me of M's bringing up what seemed like overt sexual symbols, while suggesting there's nothing there to think about, and her manner of speaking (i.e., confusing). Using this as a guide, I understood her speech as language action and her *dreams as interpsychic enactments*. I've written previously (Busch, 2009) about how the patient's use of language action—and now I would add *dreams as actions*—most often lead to the analyst's countertransference, as it is an unconscious communication from the patient first understood by the analyst's unconscious. We tend to forget that Freud (1912) spoke to this process early on when he indicated that the analyst "turn his unconscious like a receptive organ towards the transmitting unconscious of the patient" (p. 115). "The intent is to allow the patient's unconscious to impact the analyst and then observe the ensuing conscious mental and emotional experiences" (ibid., p. 116).[1]

Specifically, it was my countertransference reaction of agitated confusion and frustration, typical feelings children have when exposed to primal scene experiences, along with the association to my own likely primal experience (at the hotel), which together led me to think that what M was enacting with me was a primal scene where she was the active doer, and I was supposed to be the passive recipient. While the dream had obvious symbolic meaning, it was also dreamt to *do* something, that is, to provoke sexual images for me that would stir me up. M's lack of response to the symbols in the dream was, in part, because they were supposed *to do something, not represent something*. All of this likely repeated her early experience of being exposed to the primal scene and then having her parents act like nothing had just happened. I was now the one stimulated to think these sexual thoughts, while she was acting as if nothing sexual was in the air. The conclusion I came to was that what was going on seemed to be an example of an "interpsychic" process as described by Bolognini (2004) and Diamond (2014).

While every analysis entails the use of several if not all the stages in which the analytic drama is played out, *some* analyses in particular, and *all analyses at certain times*, are significantly characterized by qualities manifested along the interpsychic pathway. These qualities include a "doing to" the analyst, at some level, in the context of the patient's dreams, associations, transferences and the like, and requires the analyst's mind use.

(Diamond, p. 544)

I have described this manner of functioning as *language action*, and the analyst's need to use and analyze his own countertransference reactions as a way of understanding what the patient is "doing" with their language. I've mentioned previously (Busch, 2009) that children's thinking until around the age of 7 is more like action according to Piaget and Inholder (1959). This was the time when M was consistently exposed to the primal scene, so it isn't surprising that she can only defend against confusing and frightening feelings usually aroused via actions and language action.

Given the current zeitgeist of our field, it is difficult to write about dreams without referencing Bion and some of the post-Bionian views. As I mentioned in a previous publication (Busch, 2019), a discussion of a paper of mine by Claudio Eizerik led me to an exploration of Bion and the post-Bionian thinking. In terms of dreams, Grotstein (2009) made it clear that Bion had a different understanding of dreams than Freud. "In brief he believed that dreaming constitutes unconscious wakeful thinking. "It is the 'emotional thinking' that accompanies (parallels) and facilitates cognitive thinking. It includes the mentation of sense-impressions (beta-elements) into alpha-elements" (p. 741). Grotstein (2009) added, "Bion thus believes that dreaming is not only a *form* of thinking; it is of utmost importance in allowing thinking to occur". According to Ogden (2007):

I view dreaming as the most important psychoanalytic function of the mind: where there is unconscious "dream-work", there is also unconscious "understanding-work"; where there is an unconscious "dreamer who dreams the dream" (Grotstein, 2000, p. 5), there is also an unconscious "dreamer who understands the dream".

(p. 576)

In his 2007 paper, Ogden begins with the observation that:

Many patients are unable to engage in waking-dreaming in the analytic setting in the form of free association or in any other form. The author has found that 'talking-as-dreaming' has served as a form of waking-dreaming in which such patients have been able to begin to dream formerly un-dreamable experience.

(p. 575)

Given the above, it would seem like a patient who was able to have night dreams that are seemingly rich in symbols, but was unable to have waking dreams, would contradict this view of dreams by some post-Bionians. There may be elements of the post-Bionian literature that I haven't come across that might explain what I see as a contradiction between the lofty views of dream expressed by Grotstein and Bion, and M's response to her dreams.

Note

1 This point was returned to many years later by Heiman (1950) and Racker (1953), with the warning that one also has to be aware of how the analyst's own conflicts and fantasies can contribute to one's reaction, and this needs to be ruled out as part of one's self-analysis. This latter point is often left out of discussions of these papers (see Chapter).

References

Bolognini, S. (2004) Intrapsychic-Interpsychic. *International Journal of Psychoanalysis* 85:337–358.

Busch, F. (2009) "Can You Push a Camel through the Eye of a Needle?" Reflections on how the Unconscious speaks to us and its Clinical Implications. *International Journal of Psychoanalysis* 90:53–68.

Busch, F. (2019) *The Analyst's Reveries: An Exploration of Bion's Enigmatic Concept*. London: Routledge.

Diamond, M.J. (2014) Analytic Mind Use and Interpsychic Communication. *Psychoanalytic Quarterly* 83:525–563.

Freud, S. (1912) Recommendations to Physicians Practising Psycho-Analysis. *The Standard Edition of the Complete Psychological Works of Sigmund Freud* 12:109–120.

Freud, S. (1914) Remembering, Repeating and Working-Through (Further Recommendations on the Technique of Psycho-Analysis II). *S.E.* XII: 145–156.

Green, A. (2000) The Central Phobic Position. *International Journal of Psychoanalysis* 81(3):429–451.

Grotstein, J. S. (2009) Dreaming as a 'Curtain of Illusion': Revisiting the 'Royal Road' with Bion as Our Guide. *International Journal of Psychoanalysis* 90:733–752.

Ogden, T.H. (2007) On Talking-as-dreaming. *International Journal of Psychoanalysis* 88(3):575–589.

Piaget, J. and Inholder, B. (1959) *The Psychology of the Child*. New York: Basic Books.

Part II

Essays About Psychoanalysis and Psychoanalysts

13 The Gossip

A Recurring Problem in Psychoanalytic Organizations

Many analysts have had the experience I will now relate. One's analyst, supervisor, or an older analyst in a position of some authority in one's institute, or a national or international organization, tells us something, rarely flattering, about another candidate or analyst. Or it can be confidential information about the institute or other organizational politics. It is usually introduced with a statement like, "You have to keep this confidential", *while the teller is breaking a confidence.* It may also begin with, "I shouldn't be telling you this ..." It is told "in confidence" because the one telling the incident realizes, at some level, that this is not information he/she should be sharing and that they would not like this information to go out to the wider psychoanalytic community with him/her as the source. The person who hears this information (the listener) is often curious to hear this information, and *excited to have the curtain pulled back from this heretofore-secret world.* Yet the listener also knows this is information he shouldn't be hearing and feels uncomfortable with his interest and excitement. The listener is further put into a difficult situation because the one telling the information is often in a position of authority. We don't want to appear critical of this person who may have some say over our psychoanalytic career, and whom we might feel friendly towards. However, even if it is a friend or colleague of equal status, our interest and excitement over receiving "forbidden" information most often prevents us from stopping the person from telling us. Inevitably, the one who was told this "confidential" material tells someone else, without revealing the source, so that now this second person is in this uncomfortable position of receiving "forbidden" information. Inevitably the pattern continues to be repeated.

There are many variations of the scenario just mentioned, all of which have a common theme; that is, the listener is hearing information that should remain private, and is *titillating* to hear about. A colleague tells us about the boundary problems of an analyst we both know in another city that he heard about in a private conversation. A supervisor tells us about the problems of a colleague who just presented a paper at the institute, implying the colleague is primarily working out his own issues and thereby dismissing any possible worth in the paper.

DOI: 10.4324/9781032658704-16

A colleague tells us of something he heard in a Progressions Committee about candidate X. While sitting with colleagues from around the country, we are regaled with stories, told in a salacious manner, of "famous" analysts and their boundary violations. We all laugh, and only later ask each other, "What was that about?"

Although it seems to be ubiquitous in institutes, there is only one article from over 40 years ago (Olinick, 1980) devoted to gossiping in institutes, and it's specifically about analysts gossiping about *patients*. However, there are similarities in Olinick's observations to what I've just described. For example, he states,

> The one who gossips requires an interlocutor who is or will become an eager listener, one whom he can impress, titillate, or compete with in his tales of inner secrets. The listener must share in and complement the motives of the speaker.
>
> (p. 440)

Olinick goes on to describe the "gossiping couple" (p. 444).

> What is gossiped about is not necessarily related directly to the analyst's motives for the gossiping. The affective valence and investment of the gossipers may be irrelevant to the *content* of the gossip; it will reflect the needs of the gossiping couple more than it will the particular secrets of the patient.
>
> (p. 444)

These observations both broaden and are consistent with my understanding, especially his use of the word "titillate", which has the meaning of exciting someone, usually in a sexual way.

The Gossip and the Listener

Studies of gossip have pointed to its effect on social groups over time. Evolutionary biologists identified gossip as aiding social bonding in large groups. More recent studies focused on the destructive consequences of gossip in the workplace, and its role in defining power differentials between individuals.

In my experience, the essential element in the gossiping dyads I've described earlier (i.e., a senior colleague gossiping about something "I probably shouldn't be telling you") *involves a seductive invitation into the primal scene.* The listener is invited to engage in *auditory voyeurism*, as the gossip opens a door to what should remain hidden. The feeling of excitement, accompanied by the sense of discomfort, mirrors the feelings of the patients we see as adults who experienced premature sexual excitement with parents or older siblings. For the gossip, it is an unconscious enactment of forcing the other to participate in an illicit act from a position of power or authority. For the listener it is like being invited into the parental bedroom, with all the excitement and uneasiness such an invitation brings about. It is striking how rare it is that when a senior colleague says, "I probably shouldn't be saying this …", we don't stop him/her by simply saying, "Then I probably shouldn't be hearing it". Instead, we respond to our own excitement about "What's going on there behind those closed doors?" and a wish to gratify the gossip who gains satisfaction by having this secret information and letting another know he has it.

It should be no surprise then that the term gossip *originates from the bedroom at the time of childbirth.* Giving birth used to be a social (women only) event, where a pregnant woman's female relatives and neighbors would gather. As with any social gathering there was chattering, and this is where the term *gossip* came to mean talk of others. Olinick (1980) wrote about analysts who gossip regarding patients and concluded, "there is little doubt that segments or *derivatives of primal scenes are enacted* when gossips meet, both in the fact that secret actions are being gossiped about, and the gossiping is taking place as itself a piece of forbidden action" (p. 443, italics added). Kernberg (1986) described the unavoidable repetition of "primal scene" material in psychoanalytic institutes. Eissler (1993), who writes about his experience of being maligned by gossip, uses sexual metaphors to distinguish between types of gossip (e.g., soft-core gossip), without labeling it as such. I've only been able to find one example in the psychoanalytic literature (Rosenbaum and Subrin, 1963) where gossip was a primary symptom. The patient seemed to be forced into treatment when his malicious gossiping came back to haunt him. Within the treatment, the gossiping was traceable back to the patient's Oedipal collusion with the mother to eliminate rivals. "At home, he would discuss at great length with his mother the negative aspect of his father's personality and behavior" (p. 825).

A patient of mine recently told of the following incident. He was meeting with his team of consultants and had to tell them of the departure of one of their colleagues. This fellow was fired due to mismanagement of discretionary funds that might have been for self-gain. My patient felt like he wanted to tell them all the dirt about this fellow but restrained himself. Another colleague involved in the firing felt that everyone should know what happened and spilled the dirt. It was a big shock to everyone. The patient felt resentful that his colleague got to tell everyone about this supposedly private knowledge, instead of him. In short, *my patient felt deprived of being the "gossip"*. He then remembered a daydream from earlier in the day. Although he was sophisticated in "knowledge" of the unconscious, he treated this daydream as if it was something unwelcome foisted upon him, that is, like a piece of unasked-for gossip. In the daydream, he was blind but had managed to kill a large snake. He wanted his mother to take a picture of him with the snake. His thoughts went to a key early memory where he caught a small rodent in the fields behind his house, and when he proudly brought it home to show his mother, she was disgusted and told him to get rid of it. In his earlier associations, this was always associated with how his mother felt about his phallic pride. However, in the daydream, his mother would now proudly take his picture with this huge phallic equivalent. His blindness led me to think about Oedipus, while his immediate association had to do with an issue we had been working on for some time—the difficulty he had in clearly remembering what we talked about. His thoughts then went to the home he grew up in. In a memory he reported previously, he remembered that his bedroom was next to his parents', who slept with the door open. He never "knew" why, but he wouldn't go the bathroom in the middle of the night that was closest to his room, because it went past his parents' open door. Instead, he would walk all the way down a hall to the opposite end of the house.

In this brief vignette, we can see how the patient's reticence to gossip followed by his envy of his colleagues gossiping led to a daydream of his mother enjoying his phallic catch mixed with guilt, and its relationship to the primal scene.

The Analyst as Gossip

Many years ago, a colleague from another city who became a close friend, I'll call him Boris, told me of the following with great concern. He was a recent graduate from his institute, and his wife (Sally) was in analysis with a senior analyst (Dr. Y). While Sally had been helped to feel more stable early in the treatment after dealing with a family tragedy, as the analysis went on, she became concerned about Dr. Y's way of working, and shared some incidents with her husband. Sally reported that Dr. Y frequently talked about other patients and analysts, often shared events from his own life, made recommendations for movies or restaurants, or suggested they have the session while walking outside. Boris was perplexed by Dr. Ys behavior but was wary of being drawn into a transferential enactment. Further, the relational/interpersonal trend had recently swept through his institute, and Boris wondered if his wife's analyst was caught up in a method of working focused on confronting the patient with the analyst's subjectivity. However, as the behavior continued, and even increased, it seemed more and more like Dr. Y was unable to contain his thoughts and feelings from intruding into the analysis. Details of his daughter's extravagant wedding, the value of different car models, further details about mutual acquaintances, all became part of the daily sessions with what seemed like only a minimal relationship to Sally's thoughts and concerns. Boris, who knew Sally wasn't prone to manufacture facts, suggested she bring her concerns to her analyst, which she did. Rather than consider her complaints as a helpful insight into an enactment, a reflection of Sally's intrapsychic world, or any number of ways it might have led to furthering the analysis, the analyst became defensive and "explained" his behavior, using a mixture of theoretical notions and the patient's past as justifications. At this point Boris' wife felt a consultation was necessary. After telling her analyst of her decision, she went to see an analyst in another city for the consultation. With Sally's approval, Boris went to see one of the institute's "wise men", (Dr. X), who had been instrumental in starting the institute's analyst's assistance program, as well as being a leader in the field of professional ethics. Boris knew Dr. Y was a popular analyst and supervisor of candidates, but also knew several of his candidates were in some difficulty in the institute. He wondered if Dr. Y's behavior with Sally suggested an intervention from the analyst's assistance committee. Before going to Dr. X, Boris decided that he would describe the behavior of Dr. Y, without mentioning any names, so that personal loyalties might not get in the way of Dr. X's view. To Boris' surprise Dr. X said he knew of this case, named Dr. Y, and told him that Dr. Y came to him for supervision. While Dr. X agreed Dr. Y had over-stepped some lines in his work with Sally, in general he dismissed Boris' concerns with a wave of his hand and a phrase one often hears, "Oh that's just Dr. Y's way!"

While there are many disturbing elements in this example, I want to focus on the issue of "gossip". There are two types of gossip in the example I've described. There is, of course, Dr. Y sharing his ideas about other patients and analysts with his patient, while also revealing personal details about his life that seemed designed to boost his feeling of self-worth (likely indicating unresolved narcissistic issues). Further there is Dr. X sharing information with Boris that is confidential (Dr. Y's supervision with him on the analysis with Sally). It is especially noteworthy that Dr. X shares confidential information as Boris tells him about Dr. Y's problem of gossiping about patients and analytic colleagues. One can imagine Dr. X might be thinking that Boris' concerns about Dr. Y's work in the institute might be allayed by sharing that Dr. Y's been aware enough that he's sought help. However, this could have been easily done without any specifics being mentioned.

It was only in retrospect that I wondered if Boris and I had enacted a version of the gossiping couple. I was primarily aware of feeling concern for Boris and Sally when he told me what happened, and anger at Drs. X and Y for what seemed to me to be serious boundary violations. However, I also realized that, in my own mid, I tried to figure out who Drs. X and Y were, and in this way attempted to uncover a secret, another variation on the primal scene (i.e., What is going on behind these closed doors?). Another question came to mind while writing this piece ... Am I now being the gossip in relating Boris' story? Hmm!

Organizational Dynamics

As Olinick (1980) observed, "We may begin with the common observation that psychoanalysts do gossip about their patients" (p. 439). It's my impression that not many analysts know that the behavior I've described above is considered *unethical* according to the IPA Ethics Code.[1] Under the heading "Professional and General Integrity" are listed:

1. Confidentiality is one of the foundations of psychoanalytic practice. A psychoanalyst must protect the confidentiality of patient's information and documents.
2. A psychoanalyst must not be reckless or malicious as to whether they damage the reputation of any person or organization including, but not limited to, other psychoanalysts, or willfully interfere in peer review evaluations in the absence of compelling and extenuating circumstances.

Of course, most analysts are aware of the necessity to protect a patient's confidentiality. It is emphasized in every ethics course. In national and international meetings, the necessity of confidentiality is repeated before every presentation that includes clinical material. Journals are also scrupulous in protecting confidentiality. *Then why is it that the types of breaks in confidentiality of the type I note above are so readily accepted?*

There is no simple answer to this question. However, in an attempt to explore some dimensions of it, I will start with a personal example. It touches on a point made by Gabbard and Lester (1995), that institutes were slow in recognizing and enforcing boundary violations.

I had recently graduated from my institute when I observed a training analyst, known to be very strict with his patients about boundaries, in what seemed like an intimate conversation with a female friend of mine I knew to be his patient. This happened several times. I mentioned this to a colleague, who had observed similar behavior, and we both believed this had the potential to be a boundary violation. We had a psychoanalytic assistance committee at the time, which could explore such issues before they reached the ethics committee. However, I never reported it. This analyst was an important member of the institute, known to have narcissistic issues, and I was concerned that he would learn it was me who brought this matter to the assistance committee, and that it would result in the end of any advancement within the institute. While I considered the possibility that this was primarily my projection, I also believed there was enough truth to my concerns that led me to remain silent.[2] Thus, it was concern for my professional career that led me to remain silent. As we shall see in Kernberg's work, this is a common feeling amongst junior members of institute faculties.

I would suggest that one important organizational element in the reluctance to report the senior gossiping analyst or any boundary violations is the authoritarianism in institutes. In Kernberg's (1986, 1996, 2004, 2013) extensive discussions of authoritarianism in psychoanalytic institutes, he concluded that authoritarianism was a "prevalent characteristic of psychoanalytic institutes" (p. 131). This is a point emphasized by many, although not in such detail (Mitchell, 1998; F. Levine, 2003; H. Levine, 2010; Kirsner, 2009).

In a series of articles (1986, 1996, 2004, 2013) Kernberg outlined how institutes develop "power elites whose interests include maintaining the authoritarian structure and protecting their interests against changes that may challenge it" (2004, p. 108). There is an atmosphere among senior faculty of sharing secrets, of being an in-group, of "being in the know", in contrast to the out-group of junior faculty who are not training analysts and the candidates (Kernberg 1986, pp. 804–805). In Olinick's (1980) paper, he described how "the issues are varied, they are basically those of power and of being in a select group of the purportedly well-informed". Kernberg (1986) also points out that candidates as well as faculty *have to be very careful what they say about training analysts*. When describing a training analyst's reaction to criticism, he states, "The assumption that the training analyst's narcissism is healthy enough for him not to take offense is, as we well know, an illusion" (p. 804). *In short, I'm suggesting that one factor in the reluctance to report the type of ethical breakdowns I'm describing is the concern over retaliation.* Kernberg (1996) describes it as "A certain degree of paranoid fear, the counterpart of the idealization processes fostered by the training analysis" (p. 1036). This point has been emphasized by others (Malkin, 2013; Masur, 1998).

Some Final Thoughts

Olinick (1980) captured one important element of analytic gossip when he stated,

> The fulcrum of the gossiper's leverage is access to a secret that he wants to exploit with others, and that others wish to share with him. To have a secret is to have a secret power over others, even while, or perhaps because, that power continually generates anxiety and guilt. The one who gossips requires an interlocutor who is or will become an eager listener, one whom he can impress, titillate, or

compete with in his tales of inner secrets. The listener must share in and complement the motives of the speaker.

(p. 440)

What I've tried to add is the suggestion that it may not only be power that guides the gossip, but a re-enactment of a primal scene fantasy. In this the listener is forced to hear something that he knows is a secret, but is excited to have the curtain pulled back, while knowing this isn't quite right. He will most likely turn around and foist this information on a colleague. In thinking about my own experiences in this regard, and looking at the literature and the work with one patient, it seems that a re-enactment of a primal scene may be a driving force for many who "gossip".

We work in a lonely profession. The wish to talk with a colleague about all aspects of our profession can be very strong, and not only motivated by power or sexual enactments. We wish to share ideas, get advice, find out about things, and so on However, we need to be cognizant of our wish to share confidential information and its implications.

Notes

1   IPA Procedural Code on Ethics, May 2020.
2   In fact, at a later time, this analyst either removed himself or was removed from any connection with the institute. The event was shrouded in mystery, and there was never an official announcement as to what had happened.

References

Eissler, K.R. (1993) The Maligned Therapist, or Unsolved Problem of Psychoanalytic Technique. *Journal of Clinical Psychoanalysis* 2:175–217.

Gabbard, G. and Lester, E. (1995) *Boundaries, Boundary Violations, Psychoanalysis.* New York: Basic Books.

Kernberg, O.F. (1986) Institutional Problems of Psychoanalytic Education. *Journal of the American Psychoanalytic Association* 4:799–834.

Kernberg, O.F. (1996) The Analyst's Authority in the Psychoanalytic Situation. *Psychoanalytic Quarterly* 65:137–157.

Kernberg, O.F. (2004) Discussion: "Problems of Power in Psychoanalytic Institutions". *Psychoanalytic Inquiry* 24:106–121.

Kernberg, O.F. (2013) The Development of a Personal View of the Psychoanalytic Field. *Psychoanalytic Dialogues* 23:129–138.

Kirsner, D. (2009) *Unfree Associations: Inside Psychoanalytic Institute.* New York: Jason Aronson.

Levine, F.J. (2003) The Forbidden Quest and the Slippery Slope: Roots of Authoritarianism in Psychoanalysis. *Journal of the American Psychoanalytic Association* 51:203–245.

Levine, H.B. (2010) The Sins of the Fathers: Freud, Narcissistic Boundary Violations, and their Effects on the Politics of Psychoanalysis. *International Forum of Psychoanalysis* 19:43–50.

Malkin, V. (2013) *Still Practicing: The Heartaches and Joys of a Clinical Career,* by Sandra Buechler, Routledge New York, and London, 2012. *American Journal of Psychoanalysis* 73:411–413.

Masur, C. (1998) The Training Analyst System: Asset or Liability? *Journal of the American Psychoanalytic Association* 46:539–549.

Mitchell, S. (1998) The Analyst's Knowledge and Authority. *Psychoanalytic Quarterly* 67:1–31.

Olinick, S.L. (1980) The Gossiping Psychoanalyst. *International Review of Psychoanalysis* 7:439–445.

Rosenbaum, J.B. and Subrin, M. (1963) The Psychology of Gossip. *Journal of the American Psychoanalytic Association* 11:817–831.

14 The Good-Enough Discussant

Having heard over a hundred discussions of my own papers and listened to many more discussions of others' presentations, I have come to some conclusions about the role of the discussant. In my view, the *good-enough discussant*'s role should be to *start* the discussion of the *paper given*. It is one of the dictionary definitions of "discuss": *to converse or talk about* (Webster International Dictionary, 3rd Edition). The author of a paper constructs a narrative to try and further our thinking on a particular topic, that is a clinical way of working or a theoretical attempt to improve on a previously postulated idea. As the speaker has been invited to give this paper, it seems only natural that the discussion should focus on the author's narrative and the coherence of the argument used to support it. However, I often find discussants with different agendas.

In my view, the *good-enough discussant*'s role should be to *start* the discussion of the *paper given*. It is one of the dictionary definitions of "discuss": *to converse or talk about* (Webster International Dictionary, 3rd Edition).[1] The author of a paper constructs a narrative to try and further our thinking on a particular topic, that is, a clinical way of working or a theoretical attempt to improve on a previously postulated idea. As the speaker has been invited to give this paper, it seems only natural that the discussion should focus on the author's narrative and the coherence of the argument used to support it. There are a variety of ways one might approach this task, including questions about the general theme or a section of the paper; praise for the thinking of the author and comparisons to others; criticism of the concepts or arguments in the paper; an example that might shed further light or contradict the author's main point; and so on. What I'm suggesting is that while the content may vary, the *good-enough discussant*'s focus is on the paper given.

A *good-enough discussion* needn't be more than 10–15 minutes; otherwise, it can take focus away from the paper under discussion. It is wise for the discussant to remember it is our job to highlight or raise questions about the paper, not to give the definitive response to it. We are starting a discussion that will continue with comments from other discussants or the audience.

DOI: 10.4324/9781032658704-17

Writing a *good-enough discussion* is not an easy task. The discussant needs to narrow his focus in a way that is difficult to do. Most of us, when faced with a series of ideas in a paper, want to comment on all of them. We see an opportunity to expand on thoughts or questions we've had or were stimulated by the paper. In general, the *good-enough discussant* needs to put his narcissistic investment in his own ideas aside to libidinally invest in the ideas of another.

The Problematic Discussant

What Did You Think of My Most Recent Book?

This is the punchline to the joke about the author dominating conversation at a cocktail party, who finally says, "I'm sorry I'm going on about myself and I haven't heard about you. Tell me, what did you think of my most recent book?" These are the discussants that use the author's paper as a jumping-off point for their own ideas. The most egregious example of this was a discussant I heard whose discussion entailed reading a paper of his from 20 years previously. However, there are many variations on this in a less extreme form. Rather than engaging with the paper presented, the discussant presents his own ideas about the topic. The audience then has two competing papers to discuss. If the speaker cares to respond, the discussion now becomes about the discussant's paper.

The Examiner

This discussant takes as his mandate a Talmudic reading of the text, so that every line is scrutinized for its truth-value or lack thereof. The audience is forced to hear much of the paper again, with the discussant's judgments of almost every line. By the time this discussant is finished, those in the audience who are still awake have forgotten what the *author* of the paper was trying to understand.

The Clinical Example

In this situation, the discussant takes a clinical example from the paper, no matter how minute a part of the paper it might be, and gives his alternate understanding. He may attempt to relate his understanding to the paper or not. We are mostly supposed to be left with the impression of the discussant's superior clinical capacities.

The Competitor

See "The Clinical Example".

The Summarizer

This discussant spends his allotted time giving a detailed summary of what the speaker has just presented. As an audience member, one keeps hoping, in vain as it turns out, that this type of discussant will have some thought about the speaker's paper. Sometimes in hearing such a discussion it can sharpen one's views of the paper, but for the most part, it leaves the audience in a vacuous stupor.

I'll See What Comes to Mind

This discussant comes to the microphone with some small, crumpled pieces of paper, spends the first minute shuffling through these papers looking for order, and then presents a series of idle thoughts that seem to have been stimulated by the paper, but only tangentially. He continually looks back at his crumpled paper looking for the wisdom he feels he must have placed there. If he's not stopped by the moderator, the allotted time for the meeting will end on this unsatisfactory note.

Note

1 While this seems obvious, the reader will see why I raise it in later comments.

15 On Publishing

I find myself increasingly reluctant to submit what I write to psychoanalytic journals. It's my impression there have been significant changes
in reviewing papers for publication since I first started writing and
was on various editorial boards. I find the whole process of attempting to have a paper published in journals an increasingly *arduous and
unpleasant* process—not all journals, but some. Although I've published 80 articles in the psychoanalytic literature, with many translated into other languages, I've found that sometimes, when there is a
change in editor at a journal where I've previously published numerous articles, my submissions are sent back for major revisions that, to
my mind, would either change the paper to what the editor wants, or
would require re-writing the entire paper.

The first editorial board I was on was for the *Journal of the American
Psychoanalytic Association*, when Arnie Richards was the editor.
Whether it was certain things he said or imparted via his actions, I
came away with some specific ideas on how to evaluate the worth of
an article for publication. For example, an article *wasn't* to be judged
based upon the author's theoretical orientation, but rather *how clearly
she articulated her position*. It is worth mentioning that, although we
had a diverse group of reviewers on the editorial board, agreement
amongst reviewers was about 95%–98%. Clarity of exposition of an
idea seemed especially important, in that many articles submitted to
journals have an interesting idea as their basis. However, it was in the
communication and elaboration of this idea where a potentially good
article goes astray.

Another criteria promulgated by Arnie was that if two of the three
reviewers believed the paper deserved to be published, it would usually
be published. The author *might* be asked to respond to the criticisms
of the dissenting reviewer, and whatever the other reviewers brought
up. I would like to highlight this "respond to" issue, as it will come up
later, and usually meant the author was asked to explain why certain
critiques might *or might not* be relevant to his article. It might involve
changes in the article or *not*. What I want to highlight here is that this
wasn't an arduous process.[1]

DOI: 10.4324/9781032658704-18

From 1990 until around 2009, I never had a paper flat-out rejected. During this time, I published approximately 30 articles. There were often requests for some re-writing, but these were usually something quite manageable, and most often helpful. *Then things seemed to change, at least in terms of my efforts to publish.* The changes I've seen can be characterized in the following manner:

- The approach has changed from welcoming articles to asking authors to "tell us why we shouldn't reject your submission".
- Articles seem to be accepted or rejected based increasingly on basis of the theoretical interests of the editor.
- Reviewers seem less and less to be given any guidelines for reviewing articles, but instead are encouraged to follow their own thoughts (and biases).

Here are some specific examples from my own experience and those of colleagues.

Example 1: Two reviewers thought the paper should be published and had some interesting suggestions for a re-write. Yet the editor focused attention on the one negative review and wanted me to change the emphasis in my paper to highlight research (of which there was little in the field I was writing about).

Example 2: After four attempts to re-write my paper according to the editor's suggestions, the editor wrote back, starting with the thought, "We are almost there", and then had a number of *new ideas* he felt I should address. My reaction to the comment "*we* are almost there" was that the editor seemed to believe my paper was something we were co-constructing. While an editor might want to help a beginning writer craft an acceptable paper, it is still the *author's* paper, and I don't believe co-construction should be part of the editor's job description. Besides, it was easy to tell who the paper was written by via the references, and I was not an early career writer at this point.

Example 3: A paper I submitted came back to me with scathing reviews. It was clear from the reviews that the reviewers had a very different theoretical orientation than I did, and that the editor giving my paper to be evaluated by these particular reviewers almost assured negative reviews. In contrast to Arnie Richards' wish for theory-free evaluations of submitted papers, editors seem more inclined to embrace their own theoretical biases.

Example 4: A colleague described to me how an article was not even accepted for review (unheard of in my time), as it seemed to challenge the editorial board's preferred theory.

While I have published many articles since 2009, it has been most often at the *request* of a journal to make a contribution, or else I have found certain journals more accepting of my work. Along the way,

I've had to ask myself if the quality of my writing has changed since 2009. Have I become one of those writers who has a good idea, but an inadequate follow-up? I don't think so. However, obviously I'm narcissistically involved in my own ideas, so I'm likely not the best judge of my writing.

Note

1　As an aside, as far as I could tell, although Arnie had his own ideas about psychoanalysis, as far as the journal was concerned, he was theory-free in accepting articles. It is worth noting that under Arnie's editorship, the journal's readership was at an all-time high.

16 On Writing

Over the years I discovered that I writefor various reasons. I say it this way because when I started my psychoanalytic journey, I never planned to be a writer, and I didn't know what impelled me to write. At some point, I realized that I had started writing—and continued to write—in order to understand something that was puzzling me. Once I was able to find my own mind through psychoanalysis, I realized that I had many questions about *assumed wisdom*.

I found there was no better way to approach the many questions I had than writing about them. Only in writing am I able to see how an interesting idea—when put to paper—is full of vagueness, gaps in logic, or unsubstantiated speculations. Being honest with myself about the clarity of my ideas is one of the most difficult parts of writing. It is easy, sometimes, to both realize an idea needs further elaboration and say to myself, "Oh, it's good enough". Through work on editorial boards, I found that often a paper submitted to a journal has a thought-provoking idea as its premise, but the author offers fuzzy explanations or ambiguous clinical examples to support an argument. Given my own experience, it is not difficult to understand how this happens. It's always helpful to have a colleague who will be frank in her/his criticism, and I've been fortunate in this regard.

I believe that over the past 40years, I have discovered elements of psychoanalytic technique—and a Freudian theory that explains them—that are central to how psychoanalysis is curative.[1] As my understanding has developed through analytic work with patients and by reading new authors, my thinking has expanded from the ideas expressed in my first papers (1992, 1993) on technique.[2] I've found that when I present my perspective to analysts from different psychoanalytic cultures, it is well received. So, I write because I feel I have something important to offer psychoanalysts, and I keep trying to find ways to improve, elaborate, and explain it.

Though I like the craft of writing, I also enjoy the exploratory process that prepares me to write. This means combing through the literature to see what others have found. PEP has made this so much easier than it used to be. I enjoy leisurely discovering new authors who help me find a way to think through an idea, and also, those who may have

DOI: 10.4324/9781032658704-19

contradictory ideas. It can be humbling to think that I have a good idea and then find that many have already written about it. Writing takes a lot of time, especially when I'm starting a project. It helps if one enjoys roaming around in one's mind. In this sense, writing is like self-analysis.

All writers must deal with publishing. There is a narcissistic vulnerability whenever we submit our ideas for evaluation. Over the years, I have found that there are significant differences between writing a book and writing for a journal. My publishers (Routledge and Jason Aronson Press) are primarily interested in my ideas and how I plan to explain them. Journals, though interested in ideas, have often been sticklers for "scientific" presentation. Both book and journal forms have value. However, I have not had much success in in convincing journal editors that a particular critique may be misguided. I think there is an understandable dynamic in which editors feel they must support their reviewers, and reviewers' biases sometimes prevail.

In summary, I hope that I have been able to convey the pleasures and difficulties in writing. I feel fortunately that for me, the pleasures outweigh the difficulties. Isn't that what we hope for in life?

References

Busch, F. (1992) Recurring Thoughts on the Unconscious Ego Resistances. *Journal of the American Psychoanalytic Association* 40:1089–1115.

Busch, F. (1993) In the Neighborhood: Aspects of a Good Interpretation and a "Developmental Lag" in Ego Psychology. *American Psychoanalytic Association* 41(1):151–177.

Busch, F. (2014) *Creating a Psychoanalytic Mind: A Psychoanalytic Method and Theory*. London: Routledge.

Busch, F. (2015) Our Vital Profession. *International Journal of Psychoanalysis* 96(3):553–568.

Busch, F. (2016) The Search for Psychic Truth. *Psychoanalytic Quarterly* 85:339–360.

17 Teamwork

When I was young, I gravitated toward team sports, and this continued into my adult years. There was something about working together toward a common goal, and the camaraderie that developed when this occurred, that was appealing to me. I only later understood this as (partly) unconsciously driven.

I was on my way to an institute meeting on a beautiful fall day, when I found my mind drifting to a day like this some 40 years ago. It was a Saturday, the day when guys from the neighborhood would gather at the local park for an all-day basketball marathon. The players ranged in age from around 20 to 40. The rules were simple:your team would play until you lost. You would never know whom you'd be playing with; it was just whoever was next in line by virtue of arrival time, or how many people were waiting after their team lost. The process was remarkably civil, much like Londoners queuing up for a double-decker bus.

There were many playing styles in these games. You could be on a team with a really good player, but who thought he was the only player on the court. Whenever he got his hands on the ball, he would shoot it. Thus, you tended to never give him the ball unless absolutely necessary. Others would dribble the basketball forever, thinking they were like some Marcus Haynes clone, only to eventually dribble the ball off his foot and give the other team the ball. Some would love to play offense, but would only half-heartedly play defense.

On the day I was thinking about, I was teamed up in my first game of the day with two older guys I hadn't met before. It was clear from the moment we started playing that the two guys I played with believed in *teamwork*. It's a way of playing where you keep moving and passing the ball until someone has an easy shot for the basket. It's everybody on the team working toward a common goal. We won ten games in a row that day, and only stopped because we were too exhausted to continue.

I hadn't thought about this day for many years, so of course I wondered why it had come to mind just then. My thoughts went to the last institute meeting I had attended. It was another frustrating meeting where nothing was accomplished because of the multiple agendas in

DOI: 10.4324/9781032658704-20

the room. In reflecting on this, I thought of how rare it is to be in a psychoanalytic meeting where it feels like there is *teamwork*. Whether the meeting is about clinical material, education, or administration, the meeting seems to always become more about the narcissistic enhancement of individual members than anything. While narcissistic enhancement can be a great motivator, it can sink the goal of a group if it is a primary motivation of its members. It is staggering for me to realize how many committee meetings I've been part of, and I can only think of a few where we seemed to be working together towards a common goal. The first was the American Psychoanalytic Association's Committee of New Training Facilities, Chaired by David Carlson from New Haven. The second was the Board of Representatives of the IPA when Claudio Eizerik was President. The third was the first two years I was on the Educational Committee of the IPA with Shmuel Ehrlich as the Chair. In mentioning the head of the committee, it's obvious that a Chair can set a tone for or against working together. However, it is equally clear that unless the group is strong in its purpose, any individual can sabotage the goals of a leader. It is also striking how easily the members of a group can fall to the lowest common denominator once narcissistic enhancement starts to become prominent. Unfortunately, I have seen it within myself.

It is interesting to note that my experiences of teamwork occurred at the national and international level, outside of my own institutes. My experience suggests that in groups outside our institutes, we may not bring the unacknowledged agendas, envy, jealousy, and rivalries that seem to be part of every institute. I don't want to idealize what goes on at the national and international level, as I've seen the same groups that worked so well turn very ugly when a leader and some members have self-serving agendas.

18 The Troubling Problem of Authority in Institutes

Authority: An individual as a specialist in a given field who is the source of conclusive statements or testimony (Webster's Third International Dictionary, 1993).

Authoritarian: Favoring a principal of blind submission to authority (ibid.).

Often authority and authoritarianism are confused, and this may also happen with the concepts of authority and the exercise of power. *Authority* is often used interchangeably with the term *power*. However, their meanings differ: while *power* is defined as the ability to influence somebody to do something that he/she would not otherwise have done, authority *refers to a claim of legitimacy* As Kernberg (1996) noted, "Authority, in short, refers to the 'functional' aspects of the exercise of power; *it is the legitimate authority vested in leadership* and involves the requirements for carrying out leadership functions" (p. 142). Shephard and Green (2003) believe *legitimacy* is vital to the notion of authority and is the main means by which authority is distinguished from the more general concept of power. Power can be exerted by the use of force or violence. Power becomes the main vehicle by which authoritarianism is carried out.

On Knowledge

Knowledge! We have long had an ambivalent relationship with it in psychoanalysis. Who has it, who doesn't, who says who has it, and who doesn't—these issues have beleaguered us since the beginning of our history. For many years, our solution tended to be an authoritarian one, belying the anxiety behind our uncertainties. At these times, the transmission of knowledge was more like a religion than studying at a university. Holding the theoretical line of the predominant school in one's Society became the goal. Transmission of knowledge was more like idolatry. Writers in a particular tradition all quoted the same authors, and followers were supposed to read, teach, and talk from the same theoretical line. In some Societies, it is still like this.

DOI: 10.4324/9781032658704-21

Kernberg's (1986, 2000, 2004, 2006, 2007) identification and exploration of authoritarian methods was intended to open up institutes to freer exchanges of ideas. However, what seems to have happened instead is a movement toward an attack on *claims of knowledge*, what Bollas (2015) labeled the need to eradicate difference and fashion a world of common beings. It is my impression that a longer story about the transmission of knowledge in institutes lies behind our current situation, and this is where I will start.

Ambivalence Toward Knowledge

Of course, there are institutes that give a great deal of time and thought to the education of candidates, yet in the larger picture, teaching seminars have not been our strongest suit. As Roiphe (1993) points out, "Classroom teaching is an area where psychoanalytic education is often at its weakest ... too often the sum total of the didactic approach to classroom teaching consists of a solitary utterance by the analyst-teacher: 'So what did you think?' The class is then left to free associate in the ensuing analytic silence" (p. 384–385).

The tripartite system of the Eitington model has often, in reality, been a dual model. For example, a large but informal study of self-rated candidate experiences in training by a committee of the American Psychoanalytic Association (Project, 2000), showed that *seminars ranked very low on the list of what was valued in training*. A survey of recent graduates by Cabaniss et al. (2003) led to comments about seminars such as: "Classwork only counts in the negative", "Classwork has minimal influence", "Classes do not count except presentations to process classes" (p. 85). In fact, length of training cases *rather than assessment of what the candidate has learned* is the critical variable in graduation from institutes of the American Psychoanalytic Association (Cherry et al., 2004). Cabannis et al. (2003), in a study of 13 psychoanalytic institutes in this same association, found that only one Chair of progression committees felt that *classroom work was an important factor*. It is not surprising then that Skorczewski (2008) found almost nothing on the nature of pedagogy in the psychoanalytic literature devoted to education.

The most important experiences for candidates are those that had little to do with the full range of knowledge one might gain in a psychoanalytic education, but were the most personal and open to the greatest range of transferences: *personal analysis and supervision*. Evaluation by supervisors seems to be the primary method by which we gauge candidates' progress, *while performance in seminars draws little attention except if it is outrageous*. A pleasant enough person sitting almost silent through years of seminars is rarely discussed in progression committees. "But his supervisors think he's doing OK" is often a response to perceived classroom problems, although we know the transference of supervisors to supervisees is one of the most frequent but least acknowledged issues in evaluating candidates.

Given how little weight is given to classroom performance in evaluating candidates, teachers have little or no backing from institutional authority. I remember how surprised I was when a candidate in a clinical seminar, where candidates all took turns presenting clinical material, said she wouldn't present a case because she was pleased with the way she was seeing the case. However, this lack of curiosity and clinical arrogance was nothing compared to the shock I had when I brought this incident up in our education committee when discussing this candidate's work, and no-one seemed bothered by this information. Not surprisingly, this lack of reaction seemed based on the fact that "her supervisors feel she is doing well". The idea that we receive information from different sources in analytic education seems a relic from the past.

Not surprisingly, the well-documented authoritarian stance of institutes kept the questioning of educational practices at a minimum. The implicit model was of a *trade school* (Kernberg, 1986), where one learned a clearly defined skill. It was based on how to fix things, not reflecting on the underlying assumptions that go into the "fixing". This is in contrast to the psychoanalytic institute as an advanced post-doctoral program, where the goal would be, the pursuit, production and dissemination, application, and preservation of knowledge. Freud's idea that psychoanalysis is based on and includes a theory of mind seems to have been left behind in many institutes. *Fifty* years ago Bandler (1960) raised this same issue in his presidential address to the American Psychoanalytic Association when he wondered, "Perhaps the national overemphasis on training over the scientific goals of the Association is one reason why the burning ambition of our students is to become training analysts rather than contributors to the science of psychoanalysis" (p. 389).

What does it say about our views of knowledge that in many institutes, the curriculum committee is the one major committee that often isn't chaired by a training analyst? This is not to say that this committee should be chaired by a training analyst, only that at a time when it was felt all *major* committees should be chaired by a training analyst, curriculum was apparently not considered that important.

More importantly, while institutes give a lot of time and thought to who becomes a training analyst, there is far less thought given to who can supervise and even less to who can teach. For many years, it was only the training analyst who supervised and taught (as if the capacity to be a good analyst was the same as being a good supervisor and teacher). With the democratization of institutes, non-training analysts were "allowed" to teach, but they were often given the theory and other non-clinical courses, indicating to candidates (within this world-view) that it was only the clinical courses that really mattered. Never stated, but always implied, was that seminars were not an important part of analytic training.

In a study of European institutes (Target, 2001), it was reported that "in every parameter of psychoanalytic training there is a huge variability … to the point that one may wonder not only if anything goes but if the training is for the same profession". In examining the criteria for graduation, the *main focus was on supervised cases*, apparently based on supervisory recommendations. In contrast, there are few institutes where a minimal fund of knowledge about psychoanalysis is considered essential for progression. We are focused on how candidates do the work of psychoanalysis, *not how they are able to think about it*. In short, there has always been a gap between our apparent idealization of psychoanalytic knowledge and the reality of how much importance institutes gave to the acquisition of knowledge.

Perfectly fitting within this gap was the rise of post-modernism, with its emphasis on the *subjectivity of all knowledge*. Before describing the effects of this post-modern turn, I will explore the idea that *in addition to gaps between the lofty goals of Eitington and the reality of its practice, there was also a gap between our official self-perceptions and the reality of our methods of working analytically. This resulted in a false analytic identity, which many were only too glad to rid themselves of for the perceived honesty of a post-modern question of who knows anything at all.*

Trends in Teaching

There have been remarkable changes in university education over the last half-century, mostly revolving around the student as consumer. As Edmundson (2013), a Freudian scholar and an astute observer of academia, notes, the university has become a buyer's market, and "That usually means creating more comfortable, less challenging environments, places where almost no one failed, everything was enjoyable, and everyone was nice" (p. 14). As an example, in 1960, only 15 percent of grades in universities were "A"s, but now the rate is 43 percent, making "A" the most common grade (Bauerlein, 2015). Edmundson goes on to describe how classrooms remain a place for the free exchange of ideas, *the student's ideas*.

My own epiphany came in teaching a clinical seminar to candidates. I've taught this seminar in a particular way for many years at different institutes. I ask the candidates to grapple with my particular view of the psychoanalytic method, not presenting it as *the only* method, but as a method worth thinking about and incorporating. The seminars are usually lively and helpful to all of us. I am frequently challenged (in the best sense), which I find helpful to modify or clarify my thinking. Still, I consider myself an *authority* on thinking about aspects of clinical technique from my perspective. A few years ago, I was teaching an advanced group of candidates when, in the midst of a discussion, a candidate interrupted to say she liked the previous way a clinical seminar was taught, where *everyone sat around and just said what he or she thought about the case.* It was at that point I realized what had only been in the background of my mind, that a new era in psychoanalytic institutes had arrived … our *Kumbaya* moment, the era of *false democratization.* That is, we were now all the same, no-one knew anything more than anyone else, and everything was supposed to be nice. No-one needed to be taught, if indeed there was anything to be taught; rather our job had become to help candidates find his or her "own analytic voice" (Levin, 2006). Skorczewski (2008) reports on how a candidate felt demoralized in a seminar: "It made me feel like a novice who could never really understand psychoanalysis, not to mention practice it like my instructors, who are experts in the field" (p. 369). While Skorczewski takes this at face value as the result of problem teaching, which it may well have been, are we to say candidates should never feel like a novice, which, in terms of practicing psychoanalysis, they are?

While what happened in my seminar was an extreme example, there were many other pieces of information I heard at international committee meetings that reinforced the idea that this anti-authority movement, inherent in the post-modern views of psychoanalytic theory and technique, was now a growing philosophical stance in psychoanalytic organizations, *revolving around the issue of evaluation.* In a well-regarded institute in Latin America, candidates refused to be evaluated by the faculty, refused to be called candidates, and will not attend seminars of their scholarly faculty who are known to not primarily mirror the candidates' views. There are two arguments frequently heard in defense of not critiquing candidates. The first is that a candidate's feelings will be hurt. Thus, we are put in the position of trying to help candidates learn about psychoanalysis but have to act as if the candidate already knows everything there is to know. Second, in many institutes we are afraid of seriously evaluating applicants for training, or candidates in training, because who can say what psychoanalysis is? Richards (2006), in his plenary address to the American Psychoanalytic Association, says, "we can no longer be certain about how good psychoanalysis, and good psychoanalysts should be judged—or by whom" (p. 375). From this perspective, we can no longer see the value of a serious, respectful discussion of the strengths and weaknesses of a candidate with the candidate. In some institutes, as soon as someone graduates from an institute, he or she becomes a member of the faculty, whether they've had previous teaching experience or not. We don't even want to say that experience can have some role in being an effective teacher. Psychoanalytic institutes have become like those in the mythical town of Lake Woebegone, "where all the women are strong, all the men are good looking, and all the children are above average". We have become a mirror of the university environment where "Colleges have brought in hordes of counselors and Deans to make sure everything is smooth, serene, (and) unflustered" (Edmundson, 2013, p. 17).

Authoritarianism and the False Self

In his presidential speech of 1955, Ives Hendriks expressed the depths of concern within the American Psychoanalytic Association for those with different ideas, and one can see his attempts to radicalize them further by labeling them as "wild analysts".

> It is still worth while today, for those of us who incline to deplore our professional standards or to consider them constricted and arbitrary, to recall these real threats to our scientific integrity, and to the rights of patients for whom we are responsible, by the "wild analysts" and the deviationists of the '20's. If they had been accepted in ever-increasing numbers as members of the American Psychoanalytic Association then, we could not have developed our present professional strength and usefulness.
>
> (p. 564)

These "wild analysts" are amongst those who started institutes that are now independent members of the IPA from the United States or are well respected in their community. "Wild analysis" was also a code word for how the work of psychologists was depicted.

As Levine (2003) points out, this official position of the American "was marked by a series of *deceptions*" (p. 220, italics added). For example, despite public support of the American institute's position, many analysts were teaching and supervising lay analysts in institutes not in the American. Striking is that once this authoritarian protectionist attitude began to be questioned by important members of our organizations (Arlow, 1972, 1982; Kernberg, ibid.), and the stultifying effects on training were pointed out (Kernberg, 1986), many questions about how things were done rapidly emerged. Levine (2003) covered this territory in an encyclopedic review, and thus it will not be gone into here.

It is my impression that at times in our history there has been another type of deception, *self-deception*, which led to the necessity of establishing *a false analytic self* and a defensive authoritarianism to ward off the anxiety of being found out. Once the authoritarian stance was stripped away, there was an instant rebellion against those who represented the false self. Winnicott (1975) described how in a false self, *"there is not even a resting place for individual experience, and the result is a failure in the primary narcissistic state to evolve an individual. The 'individual' then develops as an extension of the shell rather than the core, and as an extension of the impinging environment"* (p. 42). A *false self* cannot teach or learn, as there is nothing to build on, nothing to integrate or grapple with. The cleverest regurgitator of the accepted self of the group becomes the new leader, and all that can be taught or learned is what the larger group needs to reinforce itself. Independent thinking is discouraged and eventually impossible.

The development of *the false analytic self* was a result, in part, of a discrepancy between what was taught as the theory of psychoanalytic technique, in contrast to the practice of psychoanalysis. Gray (1982) first pointed this out in relation to resistance analysis. Although resistance analysis was trumpeted, it was rarely practiced according to what one might expect from the Structural Model and Freud's second theory of anxiety, which was the basis for resistance analysis (Gray, 1994). Wallerstein's (1988) depiction of America dominated by the hegemony of ego psychology was accurate in some ways but *exaggerated* in others. What *we never had* was an agreed-upon clinical model utilizing basic ego-psychological principles (Busch, 1999). Looked at closely, the clinical practice of the time was dominated more by "id" psychology than ego psychology (Busch, 1999; Paniagua, 2001, 2008). Yet Wallerstein's view has been one of our enduring and complex myths, stated and restated over the years.

The issue of countertransference, at least in the United States, also serves as an example of our need to erect a false analytic self. Jacobs (1999) points out that the now landmark articles on countertransference by Winnicott (1949) and Heimann (1950), which had such a great influence in European and Latin American countries, set off alarms in the United States. Intriguingly, Jacobs suggests that it was the recent émigrés from Europe who saw these Kleinian-inspired ideas as a threat to classical analysis. In the United States, Annie Reich (1951, 1960) answered the British challenge. Jacobs writes,

> Largely because Reich's (1951) paper solidified the view that countertransference is a problem—more or less severe, depending on the circumstances—that has to be attended to, either through self-examination or further analysis, for some years in this country,

a curtain of silence descended on the topic. Since the very word, countertransference, now carried a certain stigma—presumably good analysts had little trouble with countertransference and could deal effectively with the little that they had—students were afraid to acknowledge its existence in their case presentations and clinical reports.

(p. 583)

For the most part, those trained in the United States during this time had to either shut themselves off from countertransference feelings or keep them hidden from supervisors, thus losing a valuable method of understanding patients. As Gallahorn (1993) pointed out, "the candidates are aware of counter-transference in themselves but experience it *primarily* as something bad which must be overcome rather than understood. It is seen by the candidates as evidence of their imperfection" (p. 322).

Self-deception was not simply an American problem. Rocha Barros (1995), in describing the importing of Kleinian thinking to Latin America, points to a similar problem of self-deception. He states,

it has resulted in a tendency for Latin Americans to assimilate Kleinian thought out of context and detached from its conceptual system. This fact, expressed later in the manner in which Klein's works were published in some Latin-America countries, introduced an a-historical bias in the diffusion of her ideas, which resulted from this detachment from a conceptual system and disfigured Kleinian thought.

(p. 840)

In short, our psychoanalytic history is rife with deceptions and self-deceptions, which I believe played a role in what happened next, that is, the attack on authority. The problem of deception is not defined by locale; rather it is a psychoanalytic problem.

Authoritarian Anti-Authority

For a certain time after the theory wars (Busch & Schmidt-Hellerau, (2004), which lead Holt (1985) to declare the death of metapsychology, psychoanalysis went on contenting itself with clinical theory as a frame of reference. However, it took only a few years for a second wave of attacks to be unleashed, this time against the technical implications of clinical theory. Now we are in the strange situation that clinical theory, which was thought to be *emphasized* by freeing it from its metapsychological burdens, is itself the target of an assault. We are told that

no analyst is capable of knowing another mind with any approxima-
tion of objectivity or truth, and the theory conceptualizing this mind is
regarded as outdated and indefensible. The possibility of reflecting on
countertransference instead of enacting it is disputed, interpretation is
suspect because it is said to be authoritarian, and the analyst's position
of abstinence, anonymity, and neutrality is called a fiction. The indis-
putable notion of the analyst's "ultimately unavoidable subjectivity" is
invoked as entailing the following: "*Everything* an analyst does in the
analytic situation is *based upon his or her personal psychology* ... an
analyst cannot, ultimately, know a patient's point of view; *an analyst
can only know his or her own point of view*" (Renik 1993, p. 561;
emphasis added). In its enthusiasm for the analyst's subjectivity, this
statement doesn't seem to acknowledge any professional competence.
While knowledge itself and reflection are considered outmoded, enactment, co-creation, and the term *two-person psychology* seem to be the
new magic words. Hoffman's famous recommendation of "throwing
away the 'book'" (1994) rebels against clinical theory as a frame of reference for our professional reflections. For many, *authenticity* replaced
technique based upon a theory of the mind as the primary therapeutic
agent. While there were 261 references to authenticity from 1920 to
1980 in PEP, from 1980 to the present there were 1,341 references.
However, this fight against theory ends up with what Greenberg (2001)
regretfully acknowledges as a homemade problem of relational psychoanalysis: "The attacks on the analyst's authority and expertise ...
leave many analysts feeling that they have little to offer their patients
except their desire to help" (p. 376). *Expertise has become confused
with authoritarianism.* I would agree with Rocha Barros (1995) when
he states, "In the name of a freedom of thought which values spontaneity and confuses novelty with creativity, we are in danger of producing
bizarre theories and, in short, raising barriers against thinking" (p. 839).

In a very short period of time, we seem to have moved from a
*rebellion against the authoritarianism that ruled psychoanalysis to
an authoritarian anti-authority.* Bell's (2009) discussion of the post-
modern turn in psychoanalysis characterizes this authoritarian anti-
authority well. "The apparent egalitarianism of this position, and its
opposition to absolutes is rather offset by the universalism and abso-
lutism of its own position, a tyrannical assertion that there are *no*
truths and that *all* views are equal" (p. 333). It is accompanied by a
radical subjectivity captured by that belief that words don't say anything because readers create a further text while making their own
interpretation" (p. 13). Applied to psychoanalytic technique, Power
(2001) suggests that

> With the increasing deconstruction of technical stances demonstrat-
> ing that knowledge in the analytic setting is fraught with subjectivity

and uncertainty, technique itself is under question. For many, technique is now understood to be highly context dependent, with analyst and patient essentially negotiating what is "correct technique" within each analytic dyad.

(p. 632)

Unpacking this statement would probably lead to ideas that many analysts would agree with, but as an overall statement championing the view that there is no technique beyond that subjectively negotiated between analyst and patient, *we are on that slippery slope toward technique as* subjective anarchy.

Aron (1999) wonders,

How can we say to a trainee that this is what the psychoanalytic response should be in a given situation, that this is the proper psychoanalytic intervention, based on the standard or model psychoanalytic technique, when we and the student know there are any number of other analysts and supervisors, often at the same institute, who would disagree and do things differently?

(p. 3, italics in original)

Blass (2010) gives the most convincing response.

When such questions are pervasive and prevent adopting rationally grounded positions, they are, in my view, an expression of a kind of relativism of postmodern life, which invites us to abandon rational inquiry out of fear. The fear is of error that not reason but the wish to impose one's own authority underlies one's stance, and hence the fear that voicing one's stance is a kind of attack rather than a form of dialogue. In light of this understanding the question of the legitimate authority to define is ultimately one of whether one should trust one's reason with all the dangers that this involves, or whether awareness of these dangers should lead one to remain in perpetual doubt.

(p. 91)

What is fascinating is that *psychoanalysis was post-modern before post-modernism existed.* The radical subjectivity at the heart of postmodern thinking is the very essence of psychoanalytic thinking. The idea that our view of the world is colored by unconscious fantasies, conflicts, self-other disturbances— that is, our subjectivity—has been the everyday fare of psychoanalytic practice for over a century. Through our patients' lives we learn there is no "reality", only subjective reality. However, these psychoanalytic "truths" are what the post-modernists decry. As Baudrillard (1995), a post-modernist, sees it, if post-modernism exists, it must be the characteristic of a universe where there is *no more definitions possible. Definitions have been deconstructed, destroyed.*

Derrida, the most prolific non-explainer of deconstruction, felt that a final word, or defining statement, could never be written about anything. While most people would agree that knowledge is always evolving, Derrida meant something more than that. If one looks to Derrida for some final word or a truthful proposition, then one will always be disappointed.

The differences between a *post-modern* view of psychoanalytic treatment and a *modern* view can be seen in a lively interchange between Renik (1999) and Schafer (1999). In response to an article by Schafer, Renik wonders about the absence of Schafer's subjectivity, which Renik sees as inevitable. Schafer responds by questioning why the analyst's *subjectivity* should play such an *important role in every analytic moment.*

> But why so free a play of emotion in a trained, analyzed, experienced analyst, that is to say, a prepared analyst, an analyst with a reasonably intact work ego? That analyst—I claim to be one of them—would usually be thinking about the context, manifestations, and momentary analytic usefulness of that patient's material. I see keeping that much distance as an essential part of the work of analysis.
>
> (p. 523)

Of course, the notion that an analyst could keep a certain distance from any part of his thinking is anathema to a post-modern analyst. Subjectivity, relativism, perspectivism … these are the new coins of legitimacy. Thus, Wolstein (1982) can suggest that the contents of the unconscious were culturally determined, and thus denies current psychoanalysts the opportunity "to both create and discover their own metapsychology" (p. 412). However, it doesn't seem to prevent Wolstein from suggesting his own subjective view of the unconscious as "both to create new experiences from the spontaneous, still unlived possibilities never before envisioned; and to discover old possibilities in the conditioned, still forgotten experiences already lived through" (p. 412). Such definitions raise the important question asked by Blass (2010): it may be an interesting idea, but why call it "psychoanalytic" as it seems to have little to do with the history of how the unconscious has been viewed in the field? We have tended to view as psychoanalytic any theory from a self-identified psychoanalyst, rather than from a base of psychoanalytic knowledge. As Levy (2009) pointed out, our observations of psychological functioning "represent a comprehensive, thoughtful, tested, and heuristic picture of the human condition that is as qualified as the knowledge base of a discipline as any other" (p. 1303).

Recently, all of this has been expertly discussed, pro and con, regarding the psychoanalytic method (e.g., Bell, 2009; Bromberg, 2009; Hanly, 2009 and many others before this). However, it is my impression there remains an *unacknowledged rebellion against claims of knowledge and authority with regard to psychoanalytic education.* Skorczewski (2004) even suggests the attempts to find some truths or objective points of view in the classroom is a *regression*, which "harkens back to our earliest training in classrooms that introduced us to the idea of education as a disembodied experience, a disciplining of the self in the service of the institution" (p. 493). In this we can see the influence of Derrida and the other post-modernists. Since there is no "truth" in texts, only subjective readings, educators' "need to find ways to let our students use their imagination and find their own ways, *to their own truth*" (Russo, p. 14, italics added). In such a system there are no psychoanalytic truths, like an *unconscious*, apart from one's subjectivity. Thus Levin (2006) can bitterly complain about her institute not allowing her, as a candidate, to find her *own way*, but instead her supervisors and teachers believed they had something important to teach. I would agree with Laudan's (1990) assessment of this perspective:

The displacement of the idea that facts and evidence matter by the idea that everything boils down to subjective interests and perspectives is—second only to American political campaigns—the most prominent and pernicious manifestation of anti-intellectualism in our time. (Laudan, 1990).

Conversations on Authority

There are several conversations that I think need to take place at every level of psychoanalytic organizations. The first is "Where do seminars fit within a psychoanalytic curriculum?" Within the Eitington model, we've answered this in the abstract, but not in concrete terms. In fact, as I've tried to point out in this essay, with notable exceptions, the reality is we've pretty much answered the question of the role of seminars in the negative. We don't give much time to teaching, and we don't teach well. I believe we need to emphasize the value and importance of our seminars. Many analysts may be interested in committing themselves to excellence in teaching, but we don't reward teaching. Further, we don't consider the importance of seminar performance in a candidate's progress unless it's way beyond the norm. Ultimately, as psychoanalysts, we will have to deal with an observation by Menand (2010); writing about education in the Academy, he states,

The pursuit, production and dissemination, application, and pres-
ervation of knowledge are the central activities of a civilization.
Knowledge is social memory, a connection to the past; and it is
social hope an investment in the future ... It is how we reproduce
ourselves as social beings and how we change—how we keep our
feet on the ground and our heads in the clouds.

(p. 13, italics added)

A second conversation that I believe needs to take place revolves
around the issue of defining psychoanalysis. As Blass (2010) recently
asked, "Are there certain concepts we can say define psychoanalysis?"
Indeed, is asking this question beneficial to the field? In the act of
asking this question, Blass has broken through the stifling effects of
"political correctness" to allow for a more searching dialogue. For
example, there are concepts presented in seminars that might be
helpful and therapeutic. However, a central question for our time is
whether a concept is psychoanalytic. Shall we consider the key concepts of the major "psychoanalytic schools" as essential for a treatment to be called psychoanalytic?

Another conversation, raised by Ehrlich (2006), revolves around
the place of psychoanalysis in the larger culture.

By longing for acceptance and pursuing respectability, psychoanalysis may indeed have succeeded in becoming a fixture of current
Western culture. But the price it has paid for this is enormous, and
it is not at all clear if it can survive this development. In parallel
with its healing and scientific aspects, psychoanalysis has a powerful subversive side, born out of its relatedness to the unconscious.
Psychoanalysis is therefore best suited for occupying a marginal
position, on the outer boundary of respectability and cultural recep-
tion. This is where it can thrive, and where its dualistic and subversive nature can best contribute to cultural and civilized well-being.
This is also the place where the individual subject, tormented by
feeling out of line with cultural demands and expectations, can best
be met and engaged.

(pp. 11–12)

These thoughts stand in opposition to our many outreach activities
today. We need to think about whether a watered-down version of
psychoanalysis will result in an effect opposite to what its promoters
intended.

There are certain guidelines on which psychoanalytic education
might rest to energize the next generation of analysts in thinking about
psychoanalytic thinking. Psychoanalysis was built upon a theory of
the mind, as well as a theory of treatment. The two were initially

interrelated. Yet, in our trade-school model, we have drifted into training clinicians, while the theory underlining psychoanalytic treatment has slowly faded into folklorish truism, passed down from generation to generation. This trend should be reversed. Many thoughtful faculty members and chairs of curriculum committees have tried to enhance the quality of the teaching/learning experience but often face stiff resistance. Below are some points that I've learned about and developed over the last 30 years.

1. The travel metaphor: I have always found it helpful to liken psychoanalytic education to visiting a new city for the first time. In order to get a sense of the city, one needs to take a tour of the whole city, and then go back to individual areas to investigate further. Psychoanalytic education is like the first tour through the city, while the opportunity remains to visit more areas in depth over time. In short, we need to acknowledge that we cannot teach "PSYCHOANALYSIS" in 4 or 5 years, as it as a vast, unfinished landscape that needs further exploration of what we know, as well as what isn't known.

2. It would be helpful if we conveyed to candidates that becoming a psychoanalyst is a lifelong process of learning and thinking. Many of us have had the experience of speaking with older analysts who have slowed down in their work and feel regretful because they are "just getting the hang of it". As Pine (2006) aptly put it, "Psychoanalytic knowing is a developmental process in ourselves" (-p. 4). When I graduated from my institute, a wise older colleague told me that it takes 10 years after graduation to understand what it means to be a psychoanalyst. In retrospect, I think my colleague was even short a few years. The wonderful thing about being a psychoanalyst is there are always things to learn and ways to grow. We need to think carefully about how to respectfully treat our candidates as adults, and assume that they have come to a psychoanalytic institute to learn psychoanalysis. In this context, constructive criticism is a necessary part of the learning process. Many candidates are hungry for someone to think deeply about them, and help them in their development as analysts.

3. Psychoanalytic institutes are parochial in their outlook. It enriches the candidate experience to go to national and international meetings, where they can learn about the multiple models of training from other candidates, and hear other views of psychoanalysis. One of the interesting and surprising findings of the Project 2000 study was the significance of candidate meetings with visiting speakers when they came to give a paper presentation. What it seemed to do was to expose candidates to this larger psychoanalytic world in a real sense.

Further Thoughts

1. Teaching: We need to bring dignity to the position of the faculty at our Institute. As indicated above, in many institutes, teaching is not particularly valued, nor is there a significant career path for faculty. Nothing will raise the value of teaching more than emphasizing the value of seminar learning.
    a. As is done in some institutes, applicants for teaching status should be evaluated rigorously. Those who have taught should have their teaching credentials evaluated with letters of reference. Those who haven't taught should begin by teaching in extension courses with a more senior teacher. Every applicant for teaching should meet with two members of the faculty on the curriculum committee to discuss their views on teaching. Criteria for teaching status need to be clarified and serve as a background for these discussions.
    b. A career path for teaching at institutes should be established. This might follow a path as follows: associate faculty, then faculty, then teaching analyst. A certain period of time at each level, along with consistent excellence in teaching, would be the criteria for movement from one level to the next. *Most importantly, discussions of teaching capacities need to take place.*
    c. The chair of the curriculum committee should be a teaching analyst, as a recognition of excellence in and commitment to teaching in the institute.
2. If we are serious about what it means to be a psychoanalyst, there should not be any lifetime appointments in an institute. All faculty (including teaching analysts) should be expected to participate in national meetings, local study groups, or other forms of psychoanalytic participation that indicate ongoing attempts to learn and think. What does it say that we've left the documentation of continuing education to our non-psychoanalytic professions?
3. Teaching Freud: Freud defined psychoanalysis as a theory of the mind, and most current controversies in psychoanalysis still relate to his work. Therefore, it is safe to say that one cannot define oneself as a psychoanalyst without a thorough grounding in Freud's work. A while ago there was a myth that reading Freud was not of interest to candidates. However, my experience is that Freud, taught well, can be one of the most exciting courses in the curriculum. *Taught well* is the operative term here. It takes a tremendous amount of planning, knowledge, and integrative capacities to teach Freud well.
4. Evaluating psychoanalytic knowledge is a crucial development for any psychoanalyst. Reese (2007) has made the argument for adding an epistemological perspective to the curriculum. She believes

that institutes can play a central role in teaching how to think critically and systematically about psychoanalysis. Reese lays out a philosophical basis, and curriculum additions, to foster an epistemological perspective.

> If we teach our candidates what we think constitutes and what constrains a psychoanalytic point of view, encourage them to grapple with controversies in our midst, let them know the limits of our knowledge, and help them develop the conceptual tools they need to think critically, we give them the perspective they need to be students, collaborators in learning, and creative contributors who help both to develop and to sustain the psychoanalytic enterprise.
>
> (p. 893)

5. Kernberg (2006, 2007), Auchincloss, and Michaels (2003), all of whom are concerned about the intellectual climate for spirited inquiry by candidates, suggest that a research component would invigorate such thinking. This would add another way to think about psychoanalytic hypotheses and argumentation, which would "counter the defensive use of 'authoritarianism' in psychoanalytic education that reflects both epistemological arrogance and epistemological despair with regard to psychoanalytic knowledge" (Auchinclos and Michaels, 2003, p. 400).

A final thought. There is an old Kevin Costner movie called *Field of Dreams*. In this movie, Costner is encouraged by a mythical figure from his imagination to build a beautiful baseball field in the middle of nowhere, with the incantation, "If you build it, they will come". I sometimes have the fantasy that if we re-built our institutes based upon the intellectual excitement and rigor of our heritage, indeed they will come. Not for *Training* with a capital T, but for the love of ideas.

References

Arlow, J.A. (1972). The only child. *Psychoanal. Quart.*, 41(4):507–536.

Arlow, J.A. (1982). Psychoanalytic education: A psychoanalytic perspective. *Ann. Psychoanal.*, 10:5–20.

Aron, L. (1999). Clinical choices and the relational matrix. *Psychoanal. Dialogues*, 9:1–29.

Auchincloss, E.L., Michels, R. (2003). A reassessment of psychoanalytic education: *Int. J. Psycho-Anal.*, 84:387–403.ator

Bauerlein, M. (2015). What's the point of a professor. *New York Times*, May 10, 2015.

Bandler, B. (1960). The American Psychoanalytic Association 1960. *J. Amer. Psychoanal. Assn.*, 8:389–406.

Baudrillard, J. (1995). *The Gulf war did not take place.* Sydney: Power Publications.

Bell, D. (2009). Is truth an illusion? Psychoanalysis and postmodernism. *Int. J. Psychoanal.,* 90:331–345.

Blass, R.B. (2010). Affirming 'That's not psycho-analysis!' On the value of the politically incorrect act of attempting to define the limits of our field. *Int. J. Psychoanal.,* 91:81–99.

Bollas, C. (2015). Psychoanalysis in the age of bewilderment. Key note address to the International Psychoanalytic Associating meetings. Boston, MA, USA, July, 2015.

Bromberg, P.M. (2009). Truth, human relatedness, and the analytic process: An interpersonal/relational perspective. *Int. J. Psychoanal.,* 90:347–361.

Busch, F., & Schmidt-Hellerau, C. (2004). How can we know what we need to know? Reflections on clinical judgment formation. *J. Am. Psychoanal. Assoc.,* 52:689–707.

Busch, F. (1999). *Rethinking clinical technique.* Northvale, NJ: Jason Aronson Press.

Cabaniss, D.L., Schein, J.W., Rosen, P., Roose, S.P. (2003). Candidate progression in analytic institutes: A multi-center study. *Int. J. Psycho-Anal.,* 84:77–94.

Cherry, S., Cabaniss, D.L., Forand, N., Roose, S.P. (2004). The impact of graduation from psychoanalytic training. *J. Amer. Psychoanal. Assn.,* 52:833–849.

Edmundson, M. (2013). *Why teach?* New York: Bloomsbury.

Ehrlich, S. (2006). Invited address for Freud Anniversary Symposium, Munich University, May 6, 2006.

Gallahorn, G.E. (1993). George E. Gallahorn, M.D. *J. Clin. Psychoanal.,* 2:321–323.

Gray, P. (1982). "Developmental lag" in the evolution of technique for psychoanalysis of neurotic conflict. *J. Am. Psychoanal. Assoc.,* 30:621–655.

Gray, P. (1994). *The ego and analysis of defense.* Northvale NJ: Jason Aronson Press.

Greenberg, J. (2001). The analyst's participation: A new look. *J. Am. Psychoanal. Assoc.,* 49:359–381.

Hanly, C. (1995). On facts and ideas in psychoanalysis. *Int. J. Psycho-Anal.,* 76:901–908.

Hanly, C. (2009). On truth and clinical psychoanalysis. *Int. J. Psycho-Anal.,* 90:363–373.

Heimann, P. (1950). On counter-transference. *Int. J.Psycho-Anal.,* 31:81–84.

Holt, R. R. (1985). The current status of psychoanalytic theory. *Psychoanal. Psychol.,* 2:289–315.

Jacobs, T. J. (1999) Countertransference Past And Present: A Review Of The Concept. *Int. J. Psychoanal.,* 80:575–594.

Kernberg, O.F. (1986). Institutional problems of psychoanalytic education. *J. Amer. Psychoanal. Assn.,* 34:799.

Kernberg, O.F. (2000). A concerned critique of psychoanalytic education. *Int. J. Psycho-Anal.,* 81:97–120.

Kernberg, O.F. (2004). Discussion: "-problems of power in psychoanalytic institutions. *Psychoanal. Inq.,* 24:106–121.

Kernberg, O.F. (2006). The coming changes in psychoanalytic education: Part I. *Int. J. Psycho-Anal.,* 87:1649–1673.

Kernberg, O.F. (2007). The coming changes in psychoanalytic education: Part II. *Int. J. Psycho-Anal.,* 88:183–202.

Laudan, L. (1990). *Science and relativism*. Chicago, IL: University of Chicago Press.

Levin, C. B. (2006). "That's not analytic": Theory pressure and "chaotic possibilities'in analytic training. *Psychoanal. Inq.*, 26:767–783.

Levine, F. J. (2003). The forbidden quest and the slippery slope: Roots of authoritarianism in psychoanalysis. *J. Am. Psychoanal. Assoc.*,51:203–245.

Levy, S. (2009). Psychoanalytic education then and now. *J. -Amer. Psychoanal. Assoc.*, 57:1209–1310.

Menand, L. (2010). *The marketplace of ideas*. NY: WW Norton.

Paniagua, C. (2001). The attraction of topographical technique. *Int. J. Psychoanal.*, 82:671–684.

Paniagua, C. (2008). Id analysis and technical approaches. *Psychoanal. Quart.*, 77:219–250.

Pine, F. (2006). If I knew then what I know now: theme and variations. *Psychoanal. Psychol.*, 23:1–7.

Power, D. (2001). A consideration of knowledge and authority in the case seminar. *Psychoanal. Quart.*, 70:625–653.

Rees, E. (2007). Thinking about psychoanalytic curricula: an epistemological perspective. *Psychoanal. Quart.*, 76:891–942.

Reich, A. (1951). On counter-transference. *Int. J.Psycho-Anal.*, 32: 25–31.

Reich, A. (1960). Further remarks on counter-transference. *Int. J. Psycho-Anal.*, 41: 389–395.

Renik, O. (1993). Analytic interaction: Conceptualizing technique in light of the analyst's irreducible subjectivity. *Psychoanal. Quart.*, 62:553–571.

Renik, O. (1999). Discussion of Roy Schafer's (1999) article. *Psychoanal. Psychol.*, 16:514–521.

Richards, A. D. (2006). The creation and social transmission of psychoanalytic knowledge. *J. Am. Psychoanal. Assoc.*, 54:359–378.

Rocha Barros, E.M. (1995). The problem of originality and imitation in psychoanalytic thought. *Int. J. Psycho-Anal.*, 76:835.

Roiphe, J. (1993). Some thoughts on psychoanalytic education. *J. Clin. Psychoanal.*, 2:379–387.

Schafer, R. (1999). Response to Owen Renik. *Psychoanal. Psychol.*, 16:522–527.

Shephard, J., Greene, R. (2003). *Sociology and you*. Glencoe, Ohio: McGraw-Hill.

Skorczewski, D. (2004). Questioning authority in the psychoanalytic classroom. *Psychoanal. Quart.*, 73:485–510.

Skorczewski, D. (2008). Analyst as teacher/teacher as analyst. *J. Amer. Psychoanal. Assoc.*, 56:367–390.

Target, M. (2001). Report from the EPF working party on psychoanalytic training. Presented at the European Psychoanalytic Federation. Madrid, April, 2001.

Winnicott, D. W. (1949). Hate in the counter-transference. *Int. J. Psycho-Anal.*, 30:69–74.

Winnicott, D. W. (1975). *Chapter XXIII. Clinical varieties of transference [1955-6]. Through paediatrics to psycho-analysis*. London: The International Psycho-Analytical Library.

Wolstein, B. (1982). The psychoanalytic theory of unconscious psychic experience. *Contemp. Psychoanal.*, 18:412–437.

Index